This book is dedicated to my grandfather, Eddie Rahm. Because of his words and inspiration, I became a medical doctor and have made an enduring commitment to provide care for others.

The WELLNESS PRESCRIPTION

The WELLNESS PRESCRIPTION

Your Guide to Optimum Health

DAVID H. RAHM, M.D.

Ubiquity Partners Publishing

Published by Ubiquity Partners Publishing, a division of Ubiquity Partners, LLC.

Ubiquity Partners LLC
3302 W. Miller Road, Suite 200
Garland, TX 75041
469-621-3300
www.ubiquitypartnersllc.com

To order additional copies, call 877-951-3476.

Printed in the United States of America

Cover and interior design: Erica Jennings

Cover image: Thomas J. Peterson/Photographer's Choice/Getty Images

ISBN-13: 978-0-615-27987-9

Contents

Introduction

As a practicing anesthesiologist, I have the opportunity to care for patients of all ages, sizes, physiologies, and backgrounds. Throughout the course of my career, I have seen every disease and condition imaginable.

I was trained—as many conventional physicians are—to focus on treatment rather than on prevention. However, I began to realize that so much of what ails us is self-inflicted. Personal neglect, poor dietary habits, lack of exercise, and a life of untreated stress have resulted in an increased incidence of heart disease, cancer, and numerous metabolic disorders, including diabetes and obesity.

Following a back injury I sustained several years ago, I opted for alternative treatments rather than risky surgery. I began to notice my back improving, and I quickly developed a professional interest in alternative therapies. I started exploring a variety of complementary therapies, including diets, natural medicines, and nutritional healing therapies.

Wellness soon became my full-time passion. I pursued additional training in nutrition, stress management, exercise physiology, and dietary and nutritional supplementation. I discovered the wisdom of focusing on disease prevention rather than disease treatment.

As a result, I opened The Wellness Center in 1992 and began working with patients to help them determine the best ways to optimize their health by adding, when appropriate, integrative or functional medical therapies to their prescribed conventional treatments.

This book is a catalog of the important information I have learned from a career in wellness, medicine, and disease prevention. It is designed to provide anyone with a simple guide to improving his or her health and overall wellness.

I have divided the book into three parts.

Part I. The opening section explains why our health and wellness are in decline and introduces the concept of illness versus wellness.

Part II. In this section, I provide the four elements of my prescription for optimum health and the health benefits you can expect.

These four elements are:

- ▶ Healthy, high-quality diet

- ▶ Nutritional supplements

- ▶ Exercise and fitness

- ▶ Stress management

Part III. Here, I discuss the added benefits—in addition to warding off chronic diseases—you can expect if you follow my wellness prescription.

These are:

- ▶ Enhanced brain and cognitive health

- ▶ Minimized effects of the aging process

- ▶ Improved appearance

I firmly believe that if you follow these wellness guidelines, you will live a happier, healthier life—for many years to come.

PART I
Sick and Tired

I t is paradoxical that in the modern age of medicine and nutrition, our health is spiraling downward. Cancer, obesity, cardiovascular disease, diabetes, and other chronic diseases are occurring with alarming and increasing prevalence. In today's world, we face many obstacles to achieving vibrant health and wellness. Most of them we can control, especially when following the four keys in my wellness prescription.

First, though, it is important to understand why our health is in decline. What and how we eat has changed dramatically in the last several decades. Quality has been replaced by quantity, and even our fresh whole foods—like fruits, vegetables, and grains—are not as nutritious as they were in the past.

It is also important to understand the fundamental challenges facing us, including our compromised immune system, a part of our bodies we do not think about very often, if at all. While designed to keep us well, our immune systems are often weakened and may even contribute to illness. One response from our immune system is inflammation, and it is worth an in-depth look because it often serves as a forewarning of serious problems.

Next, the book will discuss the ways in which oxidation within our bodies can cause illness and the importance of changing our attitudes to a disease-prevention mentality rather than the more popular and heavily promoted (and expensive) route—treating symptoms and illness.

1

Behind Today's Health Crisis

At the peak of the popularity of the television show *Survivor,* some 50 million television viewers sat down on their couches with a ready supply of their favorite snack foods and beverages. While many viewers were intrigued by the participants themselves, much of the show's appeal had to do with our intrigue over each character's ingenuity, instinct, and cunning to survive another day.

While the show, which was an instant success from its debut in 2000, was tailored to pique our curiosity—and keep us tuning in—I suspect our interest in the participants' ability to overcome obstacles lay much deeper. I am certain that many of us wondered—maybe not consciously—what we would do if faced with the challenges of starvation and how we would overcome the fear of the unknown.

The good news is that we are all genetically programmed to discover solutions for survival. The bad news is that these inherent abilities are dormant and are further hampered by the soft outer casings we call our bodies. Too many of us are suffering as a result.

While our genetic ancestors had to roam the plains to gather fruits and vegetables or band together to overtake a wild animal for meat, we do not have that problem in the modern world. Today, it is more likely that you will be run down by an SUV in the parking lot than you will be chased back to your cave by a woolly mammoth.

Today's dogma is ease, quickness, convenience, and quantity. We act on our cravings and impulses, not our needs. Our minds and taste buds have been reprogrammed and trained to yearn for salt, sweetness, and fat—often wolfed down as supersized bargains. And why not? In a land of plenty with a high standard of living, we gorge ourselves on the constant drumbeat of media messages. As a result, our land of plenty ranks nineteenth in the world in life expectancy.

We often opt for quantity in our lives, and because nothing is truly free, it is often at the expense of quality. Speaking of quality, we've all heard the term "quality of life," but do we really know what it means?

Those who market to us want it to mean "quantity of life"—from supersized meals to countless medications for every malady imaginable. Something bothering you? Do not feel quite right? All you need to do is ask your doctor if the colorful pill you saw advertised over and over again on TV is right for you.

Today, expediency wins out—we will worry about the consequences later, hopefully before it is too late. Many of us do not give it a second thought. A popular illusion is that medical discoveries over the past few decades have improved the quality of our lives while adding to our longevity. While that may have once been true, this is a good time for a reality check.

While it is true that human life expectancy has increased slowly but steadily over the past thousand years, we may be at the tipping point and heading in the opposite direction. In a special report appearing in the *New England Journal of Medicine* (March 17, 2005), authors Olshansky et al. state, "From our analysis of the effect of obesity on longevity, we conclude that the steady rise in life expectancy during the past two centuries may soon come to an end." In the report, the researchers propose that children and young adults may soon have a shorter life expectancy than their parents have if the obesity epidemic is left unaddressed.

Does this mean we have blunted our innate ability to survive because we prefer instant gratification? While our bodies are designed to crave adequate sustenance, are we eating ourselves to death?

The Obesity Epidemic: Cause and Effect

Today, 35 percent of adults in the United States are overweight, and another 30 percent are obese, according to data from the National Health and Nutrition Examination Survey, a division of the CDC.

Countless studies have established a direct relationship between body weight and cardiovascular disease, hypertension, type 2 diabetes, stroke, respiratory system disease, and most forms of cancer. If current trends continue, nearly 90 percent of adults will be overweight or obese by 2030. These statistics are gleaned from research at the Johns Hopkins Bloomberg School of Public Health, the Agency for Healthcare Research and Quality (AHRQ), and the University of Pennsylvania School of Medicine. They also appeared in the medical journal *Obesity* (July 2008). Researchers conducted projection analyses based on data collected over the past three decades from nationally representative surveys.

Body mass index, or BMI, is a measure that is commonly used to assess an individual's weight status. BMI is an equation that gives a numerical rating of one's health based on height and weight. As one's BMI goes up, so does his or her risk of developing weight-related diseases such as heart disease and diabetes. Current standards define adults with a BMI between 25 and 29.9 as overweight. Adults with a BMI of 30 or higher are considered obese.

Many experts tout BMI as the most accurate way to determine the effect of weight on your health. In fact, most medical research today uses BMI as an indicator of one's health status and disease risk. Both the overweight and obese are at an increased risk of developing diseases.

Where It All Begins

Many researchers believe that 90 percent of all diseases begin in the digestive tract due to improper diet, digestion, absorption, and assimilation of nutrients.

Think about these facts:

▶ Every cell, tissue, bone, gland, and organ in the body needs to be fueled and nourished by nutrients. Without proper nutrition, all components of the body are at risk for premature deterioration, resulting in disease.

► The body's natural defense mechanism against disease—the immune system—is highly dependent upon the absorption of appropriate nutrients to fuel its function. Without proper absorption of essential nutrients, the immune system is unable to ward off potential disease or to battle effectively against existing conditions.

According to a digestive health knowledge survey conducted in early 2003 by the American Gastroenterological Association and funded by the California Dried Plum Board, digestive health problems are suffered fairly equally among all age groups. Heartburn, abdominal pain, and diarrhea are almost universally suffered by thirty-six million Americans more than three times a month. Constipation, diarrhea, or nausea affects roughly fifteen million Americans more than three times a month per symptom. It does not have to be this way.

Overconsumption

There was an advertisement on TV in the 1970s featuring an overweight, sad-looking fellow sitting in front of an empty, oversized bowl. He complained to his wife and the viewing audience, "I can't believe I ate the whole thing." Alka-Seltzer ruled the commercial airwaves in those days with two other taglines: "Try it, you'll like it," and "Plop, plop, fizz, fizz—oh, what a relief it is." Plus, they had an adorable cartoon figure named "Speedy" sporting a tilted hat resembling one of the fizzing tablets.

Of course, the actor in the commercial found relief from his indigestion (and gluttony) after plopping two of the Alka-Seltzer tablets—which contained the secret ingredients baking soda and aspirin—in water. We then see our friend ready to tackle his next meal with the same unabashed zeal. The message? Eat whatever you want, whenever you want, even if your body is trying to warn you.

Fast-forward thirty years. Based on a 1999 phone survey of 1,200 people in Olmstead County, Minnesota, the *Mayo Clinic Proceedings* (February 2003 issue) concluded that few individuals in Olmstead were meeting the national recommendations for intake of fruits, vegetables, and dietary fat. Specifically, the survey found that only 16 percent of the population reported meeting standard dietary recommendations for consumption of five or more servings of fruits and/or vegetables per day and no more than 30 percent of calories from fat. Unfortunately, this is not occurring only in Minnesota.

It is all too common in our society to consume large quantities of partially hydrogenated fatty acids and processed fast foods packed with sodium and sugar. Many of the foods we eat are refined to the point that adequate levels of most nutrients vanish. It should come as no surprise that obesity, gastrointestinal ailments, and diabetes levels are skyrocketing as a result.

A study from the Centers for Disease Control and Prevention (CDC) in Atlanta, Georgia, paints an equally distressing picture. In the study, researchers found that American adults consume about 13 percent more calories than they did three decades ago, a period during which the obesity rate doubled. Is it a coincidence that this caloric intake coincides with the success of a "plop, plop, fizz, fizz" mentality?

The CDC research on food intake, based on a series of surveys, found that women ate 1,877 calories a day in 1999 to 2000, up 22 percent from 1971 to 1974. Men took in 2,618 calories a day in 1999 to 2000, up 7 percent over the same period. (NOTE: Federal healthy diet guidelines for sedentary adults recommend that most women consume about 1,600 calories a day, and men about 2,200 calories a day. Additional calories are permissible for active people.)

Carbohydrates accounted for 13 percent more of the average diet during the years 1999 to 2000 than they did from 1971 to 1974. Fat intake remained roughly the same, though it now accounts for a smaller percentage of total calories. Meanwhile, the percentage of protein in diets has dropped slightly. Other studies have found that fast food, takeout meals, larger portion sizes, and a preponderance of pizza, soft drinks, and salty snacks account for many of the extra calories people are consuming.

It is no coincidence that the rise in carbohydrate consumption has occurred as the nation's obesity rate has soared, with 30 percent of adults now considered obese—carrying around enough excess body fat to threaten their health.

But even if we try, it is increasingly difficult to get adequate nutrition from our food supply. Over time, the mineral content in our soil has been depleted. As far back as the 1950s, research about the food supply found that the variation in mineral content in several foods had already declined significantly. For example, in one study investigating tomatoes, researchers found that the amount of magnesium fell from 109 mg to 8 mg.

In addition, the way we harvest our food supply has an effect on its vitamin content. Premature picking of foods, transportation, and long-term storage can significantly cut down on the vitamin content. For example, carrots that are harvested early will have only one-half to one-third the vitamin A content they would have had if they were left to ripen fully.

Exercise and Illness

Another CDC study discovered that although people are starting to exercise more, they do not exercise at levels sufficient to have much of a health effect. In this 2002 study based on surveys in thirty-five states, the CDC researchers found that 75 percent of adults had performed some kind of physical activity unrelated to work in the previous month, up from 68 percent in 1989. The activities included running, calisthenics, golf, gardening, and walking. That is the good news. Other studies show that few people meet the minimum recommendation by the Institute of Medicine (which advises Congress), to perform physical activity for an hour a day.

It may surprise you to learn that physical fitness is intricately linked to digestive function. The digestive system is more than just the entryway for food consumption; it is also the processing and filtering system for the entire body. Not only does good digestion provide the body with much-needed nutrients, an efficient digestive system effectively converts food into energy, which translates into a better workout. Plus, a healthy digestive tract effectively supports muscle growth and repair. When we eat high-calorie food or partially hydrogenated fatty acids, we gain excess weight and our arteries begin to harden. This not only stresses our gastrointestinal tract, but also can lead to other debilitating diseases such as diabetes and heart disease.

In fact, arteriosclerosis, a general term describing any hardening and loss of elasticity of medium or large arteries, does not just affect the cardiovascular system. By natural extension, it can affect the blood supply to the digestive tract and can lead to serious symptoms with sometimes catastrophic consequences.

Diabetes mellitus can involve the entire body, including eyes, kidneys, and heart—and the digestive system is no exception. Diabetes may affect the blood vessels to the digestive system, in turn causing blood flow problems to the bowels. In addition, diabetic diarrhea is a very common condition in patients with long-standing diabetes. Patients with diabetes are also more prone to developing infections of the digestive tract.

Problems of the digestive system affect people of all ages. However, chronic digestive ailments typically appear in middle age and continue or worsen with aging. Part of the reason is that various systemic conditions become more common with age, as in the example of diabetes, which has the potential to affect the entire body.

People who are increasing the number of medications they take are also developing seemingly unrelated digestion problems. Many of the medicines prescribed for high blood pressure, for example, cause constipation, and a number of drugs for a variety of health conditions stress the liver.

Who Can We Believe?

Nearly every week, a new medical study comes out that contradicts or conflicts an earlier study. One day a study may conclude that vitamin C or E is a great supplement. Then a new study appears contradicting earlier conclusions. The end result is many of us opt for safety and avoid things that might actually do us some good. This is particularly true when it comes to natural remedies—especially nutritional supplements.

For example, a few years ago, the National Institutes of Health's (NIH) Office of Complementary Medicine trumpeted a study they sponsored, which appeared in the *New England Journal of Medicine* showing that echinacea, the second-most popular herb being sold at the time, was not effective in preventing or treating the common cold. In other words, there was no benefit in taking echinacea.

If you read or viewed any of these news reports, you would be perfectly justified in thinking that you would be wasting your money if you ever took this popular herb again. But before you discount echinacea, there are a couple of things you should know. Of the dozens of articles appearing the next day about the study, only one reported the actual dosages the subjects took (*The New York Times*). What is interesting is that neither the abstract at the *New England Journal of Medicine* site—the full article requires a paid subscription—nor the press release from the NIH's Office of Complementary Medicine revealed the dosage that study participants took, so it is difficult for the average person to gauge the effectiveness of the herb versus what they might use themselves. Could it be they did not want us to know?

Mark Blumenthal, founder and executive director of the nonprofit American Botanical Council, said in a released statement that it would have been optimal if this clinical trial had tested the echinacea preparations at more frequent and/or higher doses: "Dosage is one of the most important aspects in assessing any therapeutic agent. Many clinicians who recommend echinacea for treatment of upper respiratory tract infections related to colds and flu normally use a frequency of use and/or a total daily dose that is higher than the one used in this trial."

Here is information you should know about medical studies. Even though the NIH—with a 2004 annual budget of $28 billion divided between 27 institutes and centers—spends about as much money on research as does the pharmaceutical industry, the NIH concentrates on basic research while sponsoring only about 10 percent of clinical trials.

The U.S. Food and Drug Administration (FDA) requires clinical trials—a series of tests in humans—to show the safety and effectiveness of drugs and medical devices before they are marketed. How many clinical trials there are is unknown, because not all trials are registered with the FDA and NIH. In 2003, CenterWatch, a Boston-based unit of the Thomson Corporation, estimated that about 50,000 clinical trials were conducted worldwide, with 35,000 of them in the United States. They also estimated that approximately 3.5 million people were enrolled in U.S. trials.

Clinical trials can lead to conflicts of interest. University researchers hope for scientific breakthroughs, and medical centers want trials for both money and prestige. But clinical trials are expensive, and so drug companies are often willing to pay institutions to serve as trial sites. The temptation to skew results can be daunting.

Michael Traub, ND, past president of the American Association of Naturopathic Physicians, says there are two important points to be made about drug testing. In an article he wrote for *Bottom Line's Daily Health News* in 2005, Traub says that many people are lulled into accepting drug prescriptions because the medications have been tested on large groups of people. In reality, he says, the true test does not occur until millions of people of all ages, genders, and sizes take the medications. That is when a true measure of the side effects surfaces.

Traub, who is the director of the Lokahi Health Center of Integrated Care, also says that many people have been led to believe there is not a great deal of scientific evidence supporting complementary medications. In many cases, this is incorrect. He says that most doctors—and health reporters—only have time to peruse a few medical journals, such as the *New England Journal of Medicine* and the *Journal of the American Medical Association*, along with journals covering their medical specialty. They are unaware that there are specialty medical journals covering clinical trials of alternative therapies and that these journals are also peer reviewed.

Traub adds that many of the studies are similar in size to mainstream studies and the combination of anecdotal and observed evidence of natural medications accumulated over many years proves their efficacy and safety—or not, which is just as important.

Still, I caution you to be careful. No medication is harmless—even over-the-counter products of all types can have serious side effects if dosage or limitations are not followed. This is also true for many supplements you may decide to take without a knowledgeable health practitioner's guidance. Most important, I recommend that you always choose health-care practitioners who fully understand your specific medical needs. When in doubt, ask how the medication or supplement works and whether there are any side effects.

Busy, Busy, Busy

It seems to be a badge of honor to brag about how little sleep we get, especially in a culture where we have to appear to be busy and productive. But a lack of sleep can have dire health consequences, not the least of which is a greater risk of obesity. One study found a connection between the amount of sleep and levels of appetite-regulating hormones in the body. The findings suggest that chronic sleep deprivation could be making us fat.

Researchers have long suspected there is a link between shorter sleep time and higher body mass index, but could not explain why. Dr. Shahrad Taheri, now a senior lecturer in diabetes and endocrinology at the University of Birmingham, and colleagues at Bristol University used data from the Wisconsin Sleep Cohort, which has tracked the sleep habits of over 1,000 volunteers for 17 years.

The researchers found that people who averaged five hours of sleep instead of the recommended eight hours each night had a higher body mass index. After collecting blood samples from the volunteers, the researchers discovered that the sleep-deprived had higher levels of the hormone ghrelin in their blood. Ghrelin, which is produced in the stomach, transmits hunger signals to the brain, increasing our desire to eat.

They also discovered that while the sleep-deprived had high levels of hunger-stimulating ghrelin, they also had lower levels of leptin. Leptin is another appetite-regulating hormone produced by fat cells that sends satiation signals to the brain. The researchers concluded that the hormonal ratio of high ghrelin and low leptin was possibly encouraging the group to consume additional food. The University of Chicago's sleep laboratory has also reported similar results. Results of the study appeared in *PLoS Medicine* (December 2004).

A lack of sleep also might be contributing to the soaring levels of obesity among children, who on average are sleeping fewer hours at night than in the past. Research led by Dr. Taheri and reported in the November 2006 issue of *Archives of Disease in Childhood* shows that shorter sleep duration disturbs normal metabolism, which may contribute to obesity, insulin resistance, diabetes, and cardiovascular disease. Even two to three nights of shortened sleep can have negative effects, the researchers found.

One reason people miss their nightly need for sleep is that they are just too stressed. This is doubly dangerous because both stress and sleep deprivation can lead to a number of health problems. This issue is so important that I have devoted a later chapter to dealing with stress.

While the health challenges facing us today are immense, there is one bodily system I mentioned earlier that helps us ward off disease if—and it is a big if—it remains robust enough to do its job. It is our immune system.

2

Our Compromised Immune System

Inside each of us there is a remarkable protection mechanism called the immune system. It is designed to defend against foreign invaders, including microbes, bacteria, viruses, toxins, and parasites that are attempting to attack our bodies. No other bodily system is more important or more misunderstood than the immune system.

While most of us know that our cardiovascular system consists mainly of the heart, veins, and arteries and that the lungs are key to our respiratory needs, few of us know what—or where—our immune system is and what is does. And yet a strong, healthy immune system is our single most powerful weapon against premature aging and disease.

Virtually everyone has the genetic potential to enjoy robust health for over 100 years, yet most people's bodies begin breaking down long before. Today, our immune system constantly has to fend off far more toxins, pollutants, food additives, chemicals, and other stress factors than nature intended. Unless you constantly "nourish" your immune system properly, it remains dangerously overloaded year after year and eventually begins to malfunction.

We live in a highly toxic world. Our hunter–gatherer ancestors managed to survive in pretty rough conditions but nothing even remotely approaching those of today. While links between air and water pollution

THE IMMUNE SYSTEM'S CANCER-FIGHTING ABILITY

The Cancer Research Institute (CRI) reports that scientists have discovered that the immune system is capable of destroying malignant tumor cells. Specifically, they have found that certain antibodies that recognize tumor cells help the macrophages and the natural killer cells to do so. Additional studies of the immune system have shown that the body defends itself against cancer in much the same way that it seeks to eliminate other antigens, such as bacteria and viruses. CRI believes future studies will find ways to harness this ability, allowing the body to help itself fight cancer.

and diseases such as cancer and heart problems are well known and documented, some lesser-known pollutants may be contributing to an impaired immune system.

Many present-day chronic diseases are caused or exacerbated by our weakened immune systems, especially the autoimmune diseases in which the body's immune system attacks our own tissues. One reason for this impairment of our immune systems is the deterioration in the body's cell-to-cell communication system caused by exposure to toxins.

The immune system consists of a complex network of specialized cells that defend the body against attacks by dangerous substances that invade it, including microorganisms—germs such as bacteria, viruses, fungi, and parasites—and even cancer cells (see sidebar above). Our immune system is ever vigilant, and the battle it wages is continuous. Without an immune system, we would very quickly succumb to disease.

Combined, these "body invaders" that activate our immune systems are known as antigens. Not only are they found within or on microorganisms and malignant cells, antigens that trigger an immune system reaction include pollen and even certain foods. Responses by the body to antigens such as pollen and foods are commonly referred to as allergic reactions.

According to the American College of Allergy, Asthma, and Immunology, 1 to 2 percent of the estimated 40 to 50 million

Americans with allergies are allergic to foods or food additives. This means between 400,000 and 1 million people suffer from food allergies. In some very allergic people, a minuscule quantity of an allergenic food can produce a life-threatening reaction.

A normal, healthy immune system recognizes antigens that threaten health and, with remarkable precision and cell-to-cell communication, marshals forces to defend against and attack any "invaders."

Today, our immune systems are under greater stress than ever, with immune disorders escalating at an alarming rate. Research studies frequently report that immune system malfunction is the underlying cause of heart disease, obesity, multiple sclerosis, and cancer. Preventing disease by strengthening our immune systems is a sound strategy for ensuring good health and longevity.

Sleep and the Immune System

Before the invention of the lightbulb, the Sleep Foundation notes that people slept an average of 10 hours a night; today Americans average 6.9 hours of sleep on weeknights and 7.5 hours per night on weekends. The NIH estimates that some 70 million people in the U.S. have a sleep problem, with about 40 to 50 million adults suffering from a chronic sleep disorder. An additional 20 to 30 million have intermittent sleep-related problems related to stress, anxiety, and depression.

Research shows a direct relationship between sleep and health, meaning that:

▶ Sleep loss has a negative impact on health, including the immune system

▶ Poor health itself is a common contributor to sleep disturbances

The NIH also reports that insomnia is the most common sleep complaint reported by women and men across all stages of adulthood. For many, the problem is chronic. The NIH reports that chronic insomnia is associated with a wide range of adverse consequences, including depression, alcohol and drug abuse, difficulties with concentration and memory, and various cardiovascular, pulmonary, and gastrointestinal disorders. For example, the April 2006 issue of *Hypertension: Journal of the American Heart Association* reports that middle-aged people sleeping five or fewer hours a night have a much greater risk of developing high blood pressure.

Often a lack of sleep sets off a vicious cycle: poor sleep habits impair health, and poor health reinforces poor sleep.

INFLAMMATION AND OTHER DISEASES

While the role that inflammation plays in diseases of the heart and vascular system is well established, several other prominent conditions are also linked to a state of chronic, low-grade inflammation. For instance, research has established a direct correlation between elevated levels of C-reactive protein (CRP)—a protein, found in the blood, that increases during inflammation—and an increased rate of colon cancer. In addition, several studies indicate that elevated CRP is an important predictor for type 2 diabetes.

Additionally, metabolic syndrome, a serious condition involving several risk factors, including obesity, hypertension, and insulin resistance, is on the rise in the United States. Scientists have established a strong association between elevated CRP and the onset of metabolic syndrome.

Scientists have also found that elevated CRP is a strong indicator for macular degeneration, a leading cause of blindness. The researchers found that patients with the highest CRP levels had a 65 percent higher risk of macular degeneration than those with the lowest levels.

The following is a list of just some of the diseases thought to be caused at least in part by chronic inflammation:

- Cardiovascular disease
- Type 2 diabetes
- Cancer
- Diarrhea/inflammatory bowel disorders
- Arthritis
- Macular degeneration
- Stroke
- Fibromyalgia
- Chronic fatigue syndrome
- Lung disease
- Dementia/Alzheimer's disease
- Irritable bowel syndrome

The modern lifestyle has altered our daily living patterns, affecting our circadian rhythms. This innate biological clock regulates sleep and waking and controls the daily ups and downs of physiologic processes, including body temperature, blood pressure, and the release of hormones. Ketema Paul, PhD, assistant professor in the Morehouse School of Medicine's (MSM) Department of Anatomy and Neurobiology in Atlanta, Georgia, claims there is a relationship between our biological clocks and sleep loss. Dr. Paul says researchers are working to identify the relays through which the circadian clock "talks" to sleep regulatory mechanisms to improve not only sleep timing, but more importantly, sleep continuity, by investigating how the circadian clock arranges sleep patterns.

Dr. Paul explains that our circadian clocks set the timing that drives our daily schedules, including sleep, and is responsible for maintaining sleep continuity. When circadian timing is uncoupled from sleep regulation, sleep disturbances are the result. This helps explain why rotating shift workers and frequent travelers experiencing jet lag have trouble sleeping; their biological clocks are disrupted and out of sync.

Although new drugs are being promoted to allow us to stay awake for longer periods, such a lifestyle has a harmful impact on our health. Indeed, experimental evidence indicates that sleep disorders or malfunctioning circadian rhythms—due to jet lag and shift work, for example—are an important contributor to diseases such as:

▶ Heart disease

▶ Stroke

▶ Cancer

▶ Affective disorders

▶ Depression

In today's up-tempo, two-job, always-on-the-go world, people often forego sleep. This can be imprudent and fatal. Just as our bodies need air and nourishment to survive, without sleep, we die. Anyone who has suffered from sleep deprivation knows that the amount of sleep we get affects how full, energetic, and successful the other two-thirds of our lives can be.

But our need for sleep affects more than just our alertness. Sleep helps build and maintain a healthy immune system and, as previously mentioned, helps regulate levels of the hormones ghrelin and leptin, which play a key role in our feelings of hunger and fullness. So when we're sleep-deprived, we may feel the need to eat more, which can lead to weight gain.

One of the key responses of our immune system—inflammation—serves an important purpose: it signals that our bodies are fighting for us, and we should make note. Unfortunately, many of today's medical solutions focus on the symptoms and not the cause.

(For more information on the immune system, please see Appendix A on page 141.)

What You Should Know About Inflammation

When I injured my back and had to weigh whether or not to have surgery, my key symptoms were severe pain and inflammation.

Inflammation—something we have all dealt with, possibly after we have sprained an ankle or developed a skin rash—may be redness surrounding a splinter or swelling from a sore throat. Whatever the case, the result is usually the same: swelling, redness, and pain occur along with heat. These are all created in part by the body's inflammatory response by the immune system.

> **THE 5 CARDINAL SIGNS OF INFLAMMATION**
>
> 1. **Rubor**—redness
> 2. **Calor**—heat
> 3. **Tumor**—swelling
> 4. **Dolor**—pain
> 5. **Functio laesa**—loss of function

Inflammation is the first response of the immune system to infection or irritation and may be referred to as the innate cascade. Inflammation is characterized by the following quintet: redness *(rubor),* heat *(calor),* swelling *(tumor),* pain *(dolor),* and dysfunction of the organs involved *(functio laesa).* The first four characteristics have been

COMMON ENVIRONMENTAL TOXINS	HIDDEN SOURCES OF TOXINS
■ Vehicle exhaust	■ Some domestic cleaning fluids
■ Water pollution	■ Many toothpastes
■ Cigarette smoke	■ Alcoholic mouthwashes
■ Industrial chimney smoke	■ Many shower gels
■ Germ-laden air	■ Many shaving creams
■ Factory waste	■ Many skincare products
■ Fumes from paint and other substances	■ Many shampoos
	■ Food additives

known since ancient times and are attributed to Celsus. *Functio laesa* was added to the definition of inflammation by Rudolf Virchow in 1858.

These signs represent a response programmed into your tissue. This response is one of your body's principal defense reactions designed to anticipate, intercept, and destroy invading microorganisms. Inflammation is best appreciated by understanding your body's functioning at the level of cells and tissues.

Subsequent processes of tissue repair (healing) involve cell growth and division, cell movement and differentiation, and manufacture of extracellular material.

Inflammation is generally a valuable and necessary process. It provides a protection and repair mechanism for injury and infection within the body. And while short-lived, acute inflammation is typically beneficial; chronic low-grade inflammation can adversely affect our body's cells, tissues, and organs. In fact, inflammation is increasingly being implicated by scientists and health professionals as a major cause in a host of diseases, including heart disease, cancer, arthritis, diabetes, dementia, even macular degeneration. And a growing body of research confirms that inflammation is also at the heart of the common signs of aging: wrinkled skin, declining cognitive function, deteriorating eyesight, poor digestion, and bone loss.

For instance, research published in the journal *Circulation* showed that mononuclear cells, a key member of the body's group of white blood cells, exist in an inflammatory state in obese persons with increased risk of heart disease and diabetes.

"These cells are creating a lot of nuisance," notes one of the study's authors, Paresh Dandona. "They enter the artery and [contribute to] atherosclerosis. They activate fat cells to produce more proinflammatory factors. They interfere with insulin signaling, causing insulin resistance. They even enter the brain."

What Causes Inflammation

Many factors can contribute to low-grade inflammation. Viral and bacterial infections, stress, repeated trauma, toxins, free radical damage, and allergens are just some. Another major contributor is the high-fat, high-carb diet practiced by most North Americans. For instance, new research from the University of Buffalo indicates that meals high in sugar and fat result in the marked production of free radicals in the bloodstream, which ultimately leads to an increased inflammatory state in the body.

Not surprisingly, tobacco, alcohol, and drugs (both illicit and prescription) can also contribute to an inflammatory state. And a sedentary lifestyle contributes to inflammation (and so, too, does too much exercise—think of how you feel after a long day of yard work—your aching joints and muscles are due in part to inflammation!).

Workers with high job stress have elevated levels of one laboratory marker of inflammation, according to a study in the September 2005 issue of the *Journal of Occupational and Environmental Medicine*. The results add to earlier studies showing that increased inflammation could be the pathway by which high stress leads to an increased risk of cardiovascular disease.

Link Between Diabetes and Inflammation Discovered

Research presented at the American Heart Association Scientific Sessions in 2006 found that a high fat diet draws inflammatory cells into fat tissue, which prevents the tissue from storing the dietary fats. The fats then end up in the liver and muscle, which can cause diabetes and heart disease.

DIETING AND THE IMMUNE SYSTEM

Research has shown that yo-yo dieting—the repetitive pattern of losing and regaining of weight—may produce negative long-term effects on the immune system. However, staying at the same weight over a course of time appears to have positive effects on the immune system.

In the study, which appeared in the July 2004 issue of the *Journal of the American Dietetic Association,* researchers made two significant findings correlating immune function and weight loss. One finding showed that a woman's immune function decreased depending on the number of times she attempted to lose weight. The other finding revealed that when a woman stayed at the same weight for many years, she had higher natural-killer-cell activity, a key measurement of the immune system.

Participants included 114 overweight postmenopausal women who led sedentary lifestyles and were in good health. The women were questioned about their weight-loss history over the past twenty years. One of the requirements of the study was that the women were to remain at the same weight for three months before the study.

"Understanding this link between obesity, diet, and inflammation may help us prevent diabetes and heart disease by tailoring new therapies to block the inflammation that initiates the destructive process," writes Dr. Christie Ballantyne, cardiologist at the Methodist DeBakey Heart Center and principal investigator for the research.

Scientists have been aware of a relationship between disease risk and excess belly fat for years. They have found that "apple-shaped" people have a greater risk of heart disease, diabetes, and other illnesses than "pear-shaped" people, who store excess fat in the hips and thighs. Because too much abdominal fat can inhibit the body's response to insulin, physicians often measure waist circumference to identify patients at increased risk for these problems.

It turns out that just cutting the fat does little good. In 2004, Washington University investigators found that removing billions of abdominal fat cells with liposuction did not provide the metabolic benefits normally associated with similar amounts of fat loss induced by dieting or exercising.

Damping the Flame

Several studies suggest that certain active compounds found in fruits and vegetables—known as polyphenols—can relieve inflammation and effectively lower the risk of certain diseases because of their anti-inflammatory capability. (Please see Chapter 3 for a detailed description of polyphenols and other helpful compounds found in food.)

For instance, a 2006 review of research, published in the *Journal of Cardiovascular Pharmacology,* discussed the anti-inflammatory properties of flavanols, a type of polyphenol. The review authors state that "evidence demonstrates that some flavanols can reduce the production and effect of pro-inflammatory mediators either directly or by acting on signaling pathways."

The researchers give a strong endorsement of the idea that flavanols are a potential treatment option for inflammation-related conditions, saying "Flavanol-rich [foods] could be a potential candidate for the treatment, or possibly prevention, of the broad array of chronic diseases that are linked to dysfunctional inflammatory responses."

Help for Heart Disease

Diseases of the heart and vascular system are of particular interest to scientists when it comes to inflammation. Emerging data demonstrates that the inflammatory process causes a sequence of actions in the cardiovascular system, namely the buildup of plaque, which if allowed to progress, will lead to problems ranging from angina and high blood pressure to stroke and heart attack. Several studies now confirm the notion that inflammation can play an important role in triggering a heart attack and other events, explaining why those with a normal cholesterol level may still have a heart attack. In addition, numerous researchers have begun to rethink the causes of cardiovascular disease (CVD) and, therefore, how it should be treated.

As a result, a growing number of cardiologists are recommending routine screening for low-grade inflammation in individuals at risk of CVD by testing for C-reactive protein (CRP)—a marker for inflammation. Elevated levels of CRP can give doctors clues as to the level of inflammation within a patient and, therefore, a better chance of diagnosing and treating any possible condition.

It may seem that everything we do can contribute to inflammation. That is why it is critical that we develop smart lifestyle habits, such as increasing our consumption of inflammation-fighting foods, to minimize the effects of inflammation on our health.

One of the major causes of inflammation and other bodily stresses— believe it or not—is caused by our need to breathe oxygen, which I discuss in the next chapter.

3

Oxidation, Aging, and Disease

We need oxygen to live, but it can also damage our bodies. We see the results of oxidation all around us: apples turn brown, butter and oil turn rancid, and iron gates creak and bend at their hinges. These examples pale in comparison to what these unstable molecules can do inside our bodies.

Free radicals, which are products of normal cell processes, are aggressive, charged molecules that damage healthy cells by stealing electrons. Free radicals occur naturally, and our body is designed to deal with a normal level of oxidation, but when we are exposed to unhealthy levels of free radicals through pollution, smoking, high-fat diets, and excessive stress, our compensatory mechanisms can become overwhelmed.

In the body, oxidative reactions of many kinds occur as a result of exposure to environmental toxins. In the air we breathe and the water we drink, we are exposed to as many as 60,000 chemical toxins.

Another way of describing free radical damage is oxidative stress, a general term used to describe damage, caused by oxidation, in a cell, tissue, or organ. It is one of the primary causes of immune weakness or dysfunction. This damage can affect a specific molecule or the entire organism.

Free radicals wreak havoc within our bodies without detection. They reprogram cells in a way that eventually can lead to cell decay and cell death.

If left unchecked, free radicals are believed to cause wrinkles and thin skin, cancer and cardiovascular problems, tooth decay, rheumatoid arthritis, and irritable bowel syndrome.

(For more information on free radicals, please see Appendix B on page 149.)

Oxidative stress has been linked to premature aging because oxidative damage causes a net stress on normal body functions, leading to a gradual loss of vital physiological functions later in life. It has also been cited as a performance-limiting factor in physical activity.

The level of oxidative stress depends on an individual's genetics, as well as the environment and a person's lifestyle. Unfortunately, under present-day conditions, many people are exposed to an abnormally high level of oxidative stress that could increase their probability of early incidence of decline in optimum body functions.

A Continual Balancing Act

Our bodies are constantly trying to achieve a balance between the rate at which oxidative damage occurs and the rate it is efficiently repaired and removed. The rate at which damage is caused is determined by how fast reactive oxygen is generated and then counteracted by defense agents called antioxidants. The rate at which damage is repaired is dependent on the availability and level of free radical neutralizing antioxidants.

On a small scale, this problem is manageable because free radicals are considered a natural byproduct of normal cellular metabolism. However, the average person is exposed to billions of free radicals per day and thousands of attacks each hour. In fact, scientists estimate that between 1 and 3 percent of daily oxygen intake results in free radical production.

Oxidative reactions also occur as a result of normal metabolism in the body, when nutrients are absorbed and used for energy, growth, and repair. Like many biological processes, the metabolism offers a system of tradeoffs: while the metabolism is essential to life, it also generates toxic waste products and gives rise to reactive oxygen species (ROS).

DISEASES THAT MAY BE CAUSED BY OXIDATIVE STRESS

- Alzheimer's disease
- Autoimmune diseases
- Cancer
- Cardiovascular disease
- Diabetes
- Iron overload
- Macular degeneration

- Multiple sclerosis
- Muscular dystrophy
- Pancreatitis
- Parkinson's disease
- Rheumatoid arthritis
- Segmental progeria disorders
  (premature aging in children)

There are many different sources that generate these potentially dangerous ROSs. Most result as by-products of normal metabolic processes internally, such as energy generation from mitochondria (the part of the cell that converts nutrients into energy as well as performs many other specialized tasks) or detoxification in the liver's enzyme system. Other external sources include exposure to cigarette smoke; environmental pollutants such as emissions from automobiles and industries; excessive alcohol consumption; asbestos; exposure to ionizing radiation; and bacterial, fungal, or viral infections.

Perhaps the most deadly aspect of free radical damage is the fact that its effects are not felt immediately, but rather, they accumulate over time. Medical science now regards oxidation as a primary cause of degeneration and aging, and many scientists believe that aging is actually the result of several years' worth of oxidative damage. The resulting cumulative effects of cellular instability can cause serious cellular health effects, sometimes in the form of DNA damage and sometimes outright cell death.

Damaged or mutated cells may replicate incorrectly or not at all, leading to larger problems. Also, repeated injury to cells and tissues can produce inflammation. As I explained earlier, inflammation is now widely implicated in a number of aging-related diseases.

The terms "free radical" and "antioxidant" are becoming commonplace in medical circles and media reports. This is because there is a growing body of evidence that they play a significant role in chronic disease, including two of the biggest killers: cancer and heart disease.

Research studies link oxidation and free radicals to possibly 85 percent of debilitating diseases. These include Alzheimer's disease, coronary artery disease, strokes, tumors, cataracts, skin and other cancers, arthritis, lung disease, and, as mentioned earlier, premature aging.

The good news is that study after study reveal that even modest antioxidant intake yields potentially significant results in preventing disease and promoting overall health. Despite this, the diets of most Americans do not contain even the minimum amount of antioxidants necessary for protection. On the other hand, savvy people are turning to foods and supplements with strong antioxidant content to provide additional health support. They recognize that antioxidants help capture and neutralize free radicals, which may reduce and help prevent some of the damage caused by these adversaries of the body.

Living in a Polluted World

Some chemical agents are toxic in quantities almost too small to be detected. In addition, we are subjected to a variety of chemical food additives such as preservatives, artificial colors, flavors, emulsifiers, lubricants, bleaching agents, flavor enhancers, and synthetic sweeteners. Despite reassurances from the industry and the FDA, no one is certain what the long-term effects of these additives will have on the human body.

As already mentioned, a chief cause of oxidative damage is pollution. Consider these two recent studies:

One large research study found that women breathing polluted city air were at increased risk of heart attack and stroke. The study involved almost 66,000 women between age 50 and 79, who were monitored for nine years as part of the Women's Health Initiative, a major U.S. investigation into the causes of heart disease in women.

The results, appearing in the February 2007 issue of the *New England Journal of Medicine*, suggest that, for older women at least, fine particulates in the air are far more hazardous than previously thought. In the study, pollution was assessed by the average number of particulates, which ranged from 4 micrograms to almost 20 micrograms per cubic meter of air. The risk increased by 76 percent with each 10 microgram increase in particulates. For women living in cities, however, the risk more than doubled (to 128 percent) with each increase in particulate level.

A previous investigation by the American Cancer Study found a 12 percent increased risk of cardiovascular heart disease with each 10 microgram increase in particulates. The study was conducted among men and women across a range of ages. An unanswered question posed by the *New England Journal of Medicine* study is whether women in general, or this particular group of women, are unusually susceptible.

Pollution also adversely affects children. A study in the medical journal *The Lancet* (December 16, 2006) points out that exposure to industrial chemicals in the environment can damage the brain during fetal development and early childhood, leading to neurodevelopmental disorders, including autism, attention deficit disorder, and mental retardation.

A handful of studies published in the last ten years suggest that free radicals may also contribute to chronic pain. Left unchecked, free radicals build up in the body and can further damage already injured tissue. Other studies, including those by Robert Stephens, a professor of physiology and cell biology at Ohio State University, suggest that antioxidants may fight chronic pain by helping the body to break down free radicals.

Ounces of Protection

Lester Packer, PhD, professor and senior researcher at the University of California at Berkeley, says there are literally thousands of studies confirming that antioxidants can help prevent numerous diseases and that they not only enhance life but, in all probability, extend life. There is abundant evidence that Dr. Packer is correct. At the National Library of Medicine and National Institutes of Health's Web site, its PubMed search engine returns more than 30,000 hits when searching the phrase "antioxidants and disease."

Packer says the public's increasing interest in healthy lifestyles and healthy aging has led to heightened awareness of antioxidant food supplements. "The development of technologies for the study of free radicals and antioxidants has led to many new discoveries," he writes in his popular book, *Antioxidant Food Supplements in Human Health* (Academic Press, 1999). "For example, it is now known that antioxidants modulate oxygen and nitrogen free radicals, which are important in cell signaling, in regulation of metabolism, and in pathophysiological processes."

Free radical damage is probably the best-known feature of oxidative stress. You have seen free radicals in action: when you cut an apple, the white flesh turns brown because of free radicals. However, if you put lemon juice on the apple when it is cut, you will witness an antioxidant blocking the potential free radical damage.

It is true that free radicals also come from good things such as exercise, which increases our oxygen use. "Endurance exercise can increase oxygen utilization from ten to twenty times over the resting state," reports an article on Rice University's Web site (www.rice.edu). "This greatly increases the generation of free radicals, prompting concern about enhanced damage to muscles and other tissues."

Fortunately, our bodies have a defense system against free radical damage—antioxidants. Although this has already been covered, it is worth repeating: Antioxidants neutralize free radicals. While our bodies continuously produce free radicals, healthy tissues negate these damaging substances and keep their levels in check. It is when free radical production somehow exceeds the body's natural defenses that problems occur, and a lifetime of oxidative stress can lead to the general cellular deterioration associated with aging and degenerative diseases.

Antioxidants include, but are not limited to, vitamins A, C, and E; superoxide dismutase (SOD); beta-carotene; glutathione; and the minerals selenium and zinc.

Many antioxidants from edible plants are known as carotenoids or flavonoids. Carotenoids offer protection for the fat-containing skin layers. Carotenoids also enhance the activity of other fat-soluble antioxidants such as vitamins A and E and coenzyme Q10 (CoQ_{10}). The most common carotenoids include lycopene, beta-carotene, and lutein.

Free Radicals and Bone Health

Every year, 500,000 American women suffer at least one fracture of the vertebrae, and 300,000 sustain hip fractures related to osteoporosis, the thinning and weakening of bones. The good news is that research suggests that taking antioxidants may prevent bone loss in menopausal women.

While levels of calcium, vitamin D, exercise, and sunlight exposure are key factors affecting bone health, other factors, according to the National Institute of Health, including pregnancy, nursing, immobility, and low estrogen levels, may also weaken bones. Like the rest of the body, bones are living tissues constantly undergoing a cycle of breakdown and regeneration. As women age, the breakdown of cells occurs at a faster rate than the body can rebuild and replace them, causing the bone tissue to thin and weaken.

Researchers believe that because free radical damage can hasten this cycle, perhaps antioxidants can offset or reverse this effect. While more research is needed to investigate this link, studies so far show promise in alleviating this all-too-prevalent risk for women.

Nutrients from Plants

Densely colored plant foods contain phytochemicals. The words "phytochemical" and "phytonutrient" are used interchangeably and refer to a wide variety of compounds produced by plants. They are found in fruits, vegetables, beans, grains, and other plants. Scientists have identified thousands of phytochemicals, although only a small fraction have been studied closely. Some of the more commonly known phytochemicals include beta-carotene, ascorbic acid (vitamin C), folic acid, and vitamin E.

Phytochemicals can have antioxidant or hormone-like actions, and studies show that diets rich in fruits, vegetables, and whole grains may reduce the risk of many diseases. Researchers are investigating a variety of compounds in these foods that may cause these beneficial effects.

The American Cancer Society says that phytochemicals may prevent and treat many health conditions, possibly cancer, heart disease, diabetes, and high blood pressure. There is evidence that phytochemicals may help prevent the formation of potential cancer-causing substances known as carcinogens, block the action of the carcinogens on their target organs or tissue once they do form, and aid cells in suppressing the development of cancer. Many experts say people who eat more fruits, vegetables, and other foods from plants that contain phytochemicals reduce their risk of cancer significantly.

The Power of Polyphenols, Flavonoids, and Anthocyanins

A major group of phytochemicals are known as polyphenols—a group of plant compounds that provide much of the flavor, color, and taste to fruits, vegetables, seeds, and other parts of the plants. These biologically active compounds have been shown to enhance health and have been credited with reducing the risk of cardiovascular disease, cancer, and other diseases due to their antioxidant, antibacterial, anti-inflammatory, and anti-allergenic properties.

Polyphenols include a large subgroup of chemicals called flavonoids—plant chemicals found in a broad range of fruits, grains, and vegetables that act as antioxidants. Also known as bioflavonoids or flavones, these compounds are also being studied to find out whether they can prevent chronic diseases such as cancer and heart disease.

Anthocyanins (from the Greek words meaning "flower" and "blue") are plant pigments that are almost exclusively responsible for the red, blue, and purple colors in fruits. Anthocyanins contribute greatly to the antioxidant properties of certain foods and may protect many body systems.

Eaten in large amounts by primitive humans, anthocyanins are found in many colorful fruits, especially berries. The acai berry from Brazil has the highest known level of anthocyanins.

Anthocyanins have some of the strongest physiological effects of any plant compounds, and studies show they may help people ward off many health problems, including heart disease and diabetes. For example, it is believed their anti-inflammatory properties help protect collagen, the nervous system, and blood vessels from oxidative damage. As a result, they are believed to help slow many aging processes.

Our bodies have an amazing capacity for self-correction and healing. Even though the body is the most sophisticated machine on Earth, like anything, it breaks down when abused. It does not have to be this way.

4

Wellness vs. Illness: The Road to Optimum Health

U p to this point, I have focused much attention on the environmental and behavioral factors that I believe are the root cause of many chronic conditions prevalent in our society today. However, much of the damage we have inflicted on ourselves through carelessness and neglect *can* be reversed. And here's the best part: it is easier than you think.

The key is to make your health a priority by caring for yourself as much (or more) as you do the other things you value.

With a little effort, you can

- ▶ Maintain a healthy weight

- ▶ Improve your cardiovascular function

- ▶ Significantly lower your risk of cancer

- ▶ Avoid the pain of arthritis

- ▶ Reverse type 2 diabetes

- ▶ Live a longer, healthier life

One key, of course, is to get started now.

Wellness Defined

Wellness requires a change in attitude about our health. Wellness must be proactive, not passive. The goal of wellness is to do all we can—physically and mentally—to ward off illness. It really does not require much effort—especially if you consider the payoff.

The four areas I teach my patients to focus on are as follows:

▶ Sound nutrition

▶ Nutritional supplementation (where necessary)

▶ Exercise

▶ Stress reduction

Wellness Synergy

When we do eat well, we increase our ability to perform better, and our mental state improves. This newfound attitude often prompts us to take it a step further, and we are more likely to exercise. Regular exercise helps us digest and absorb our nutrients and also helps clear our brains while reducing stress and improving our attitude. When we include stress management, our eating habits and digestion improve.

As our strength and endurance improve, our nutritionally supplied muscles improve our exercise, which enhances our appearance. When we feel more confident in our appearance, our outlook improves along with our zest for life and activity, and we look forward to a high-quality meal, a long run or walk, or a simple walk outdoors for some fresh air.

But here is an important point to remember: we must adopt all of the factors. The four wellness factors are synergistic, and if we neglect one of the links, the others are not nearly as effective. For example, good nutrition without exercise reduces the benefits of sound eating and vice versa. Likewise, if we do not deal with our stress—through diet and exercise—our eating routine suffers. For some people, stress causes them to eat too little, while others eat too much. For nearly everyone, stress causes us to eat the wrong foods, creating a vicious cycle and diminishing our ability to deal with stress.

Here is something else to consider. We are a self-contained and interdependent organism. All of our internal organs and systems are interrelated. We need a strong heart to pump well-nourished blood to our other organs (including our skin), and we need a well-functioning liver and kidneys to filter out impurities, which helps boost the performance of our cardiovascular system and immune system. We also need a strong respiratory system to absorb oxygen to power our blood and to strengthen our heart and other muscles.

But wellness must begin somewhere. Let us start by facing some realities about the world in which we live.

The Road to Illness

If you believe the adage "you are what you eat" (and you should), consider the history of food processing, delivery, and storage.

Beginning ten thousand years ago, ancient man began domesticating animals and started rudimentary farming. Prior to that, people were hunter–gatherers. (More on this in the next chapter.)

In the ensuing millennia, farming and herding techniques evolved, but it was not until the twentieth century that technology caused dramatic changes in food "processing" and, as a result, eating habits. For example, canning, freezing, packaging, and refrigeration technology lengthened product storage and shelf life. Then new plant and animal hybrids, along with petrochemical fertilizers and pesticides, were developed to create bigger and thicker-skinned vegetables, and antibiotics and hormones were introduced to bigger and faster-growing, tightly penned, and highly stressed animals. Yields increased, and foods became available to larger numbers of people as food prices declined.

Changes in production systems also brought alterations in food composition. Meat from animals raised in confined feedlots has significantly higher ratios of omega-6 to omega-3 fatty acids than their pasture-fed or free-range counterparts. Also, a 2006 report of forty-three garden crops, based on USDA data, noted a significant decline in protein, calcium, iron, phosphorus, riboflavin, and ascorbic acid over the past fifty years, with no decline in fat or carbohydrate.

With this much food being produced—one estimate states that the U.S. food industry produces between two and three times the number of food calories recommended for every man, woman, and child—it is no wonder that the resulting highly processed food that is calorie rich and nutrient poor is so heavily promoted, especially to children.

From 1970 to 2003, the average caloric intake per person per day increased from 2,234 to 2,757. Since 1999, annual per-person consumption of fats and oils has increased by 78 percent; and in one study, subjects overwhelmingly indicated that their favorite vegetable was french fries. With the dramatic increase in fried foods in the fast-food industry, it should come as no surprise that the incidence of heart disease and diabetes has also rapidly increased.

Let us look a little closer at a few of these recent "health" trends.

Overweight and Obesity

Excess weight is not actually a disease, but it does increase the risk of hypertension, type 2 diabetes, an abnormal lipid profile, coronary heart disease, stroke, gall bladder disease, some cancers (endometrial, breast, colon), sleep apnea, osteoarthritis, and Alzheimer's disease. In many people, it also increases the levels of inflammation and oxidative stress. For these reasons, trends in these conditions are highly relevant to disease patterns in human populations.

Diabetes

According to the CDC, type 2 diabetes, frequently associated with aging, has become a significant and growing problem because of obesity—even among children. It is estimated that more than 20 million Americans are currently diabetic, one-third of whom do not realize they have the disease. Because obesity and diabetes often go hand in hand, a new term has been coined to describe this occurrence: diabesity®.

Cardiovascular Disease

Cardiovascular disease and its associated risk factors are increasingly recognized as variables for both Alzheimer's disease and vascular dementia.

(Note: A risk factor is a variable associated with an increased risk of disease or infection. Risk factors are correlational and not necessarily causal because correlation does not imply causation.) A sharp upturn in the incidence of cardiovascular disease during the middle of the twentieth century led to considerable research into its origins and measures to prevent it. Declines in deaths from cardiovascular disease during the past 25 years are due to a combination of factors, including early detection, smoking reduction, blood pressure control, dietary knowledge, and improvements in medical care, including emergency management. Heart disease, however, remains the leading cause of death in men and women in the United States.

Hypertension

Although data gaps make it difficult to determine changes in prevalence over many decades, evidence from the CDC concludes that age-adjusted hypertension increased in the U.S. population during the years 1988–2000. For example, from 2001 to 2004, 30 percent of men and 33 percent of women 45 to 54 years of age had hypertension.

Hypertension is the most common diagnosis made in the elderly. The incidence of hypertension increases with age. In one of the largest and longest studies of its kind, the Framingham Heart Study, it was noted that individuals with normal blood pressure at age 55 have a 90 percent lifetime risk for developing hypertension. In other words, a 55-year-old person has a 90 percent likelihood of developing hypertension in his or her lifetime, according to a study appearing in the *Journal of the American Medical Association* in 2002.

Modern-Day Diets Beget Modern-Day Diseases

Sufferers of chronic fatigue syndrome (CFS) often live in a limbo of ill health marked by severe fatigue with little or no substantive medical help. Despite a host of advances in treating many diseases, CFS is one of modern society's "mystery "ailments, lacking definitive causes and, even more importantly, definitive cures.

Besides CFS, fibromyalgia—which can cause widespread body pain and range from an aggravation to a disabling affliction—is also in this category. While CFS and fibromyalgia are different disorders, they have much in common. Besides fatigue, both cause sleep disturbances, immune system dysfunction, and psychological depression. Those with CFS often demonstrate the tender points of fibromyalgia. Common symptoms include pain, tenderness, and stiffness in muscles, tendon insertions, and soft tissue structures.

Although accurate numbers are not available for how widespread CFS is, because definitive diagnosis is more difficult, CFS mainly affects middle-aged females, with a peak age of onset of 20 to 40 years. Even though these disorders affect several million people each year, medical management and treatment consist mainly of education, relief of discomfort, and improvement of quality of sleep, exercise, and emotional balance. It is not unusual for people with chronic body-wide pain and fatigue to be diagnosed with both fibromyalgia and CFS.

Researchers do not know for sure when modern disorders like CFS and fibromyalgia first developed. But there is reason to believe our hunter–gatherer ancestors never suffered from many of the illnesses that plague modern humans. One possible explanation is that our food supply, in addition to often being loaded with toxins such as pesticides, is depleted of phytochemicals and other nutrients. For example, even if you are eating a reasonably healthy diet rich in vegetables and fruits, ounce-for-ounce you are not getting the nutrition you would have received from the same food fifty years ago. It takes two servings of broccoli in 2006 to give you the same amount of vitamin A you would have taken in from one serving of broccoli in 1951.

What is more, anthropologists and nutritionists have long known that we are not eating the foods our bodies were designed to thrive on, and, due to the abundance and availability, our earliest ancestors ate nutrient-dense, totally unrefined foods. Many scientists conclude that it is entirely possible that our ancestors received the nutrients they needed from food each day—enough to cope with the conditions of their time. However, that world no longer exists, and the foods we eat today provide much less nutrition—including health-critical nutrients—than most people need.

While there is not yet a specific cause for these modern "mystery" maladies, including fibromyalgia and CFS, they may all involve aspects of the body that are out of balance and functioning improperly. For the fatigue from which CFS and fibromyalgia patients suffer, high-quality nutrients have been shown to increase endurance and to boost stamina. Because we are learning more about the importance of dietary ingredients for regulating the immune, nervous, and muscular systems as well as cell-to-cell communications in general, it is not surprising that the biological activities of such nutritional elements are critical for maintaining the health of these systems.

Bottom line: The symptoms of CFS and fibromyalgia could be caused by one or more toxic or infectious insults affecting the immune system and resulting in changes in the body's normal processes on a cellular level.

It seems that we are getting further and further away from tapping our inherent desire and abilities not just to survive, but to thrive.

The Path to Wellness

I recommend a nutritional plan that incorporates some basic principles, which I can summarize in few words—a diet focused on plenty of fruits and vegetables combined with high-quality lean meats. It is that simple. And I will talk about it in greater detail in the next section of the book.

For now, I want to try to convince you that by adopting a lifestyle that incorporates simple and sound principles, we can overcome many of the health risks we face.

Who Can We Trust?

Western medicine, also known as "modern medicine," or "conventional medicine," is what most of us experience when we visit our doctors. There's another term—allopathic—to describe this type of medicine, but it is seldom used by MDs because it is a bit of a slur. Derived from Greek, its close translation is "opposite suffering." The term is credited to Samuel Hahnemann, an early proponent of homeopathy. Homeopathy focuses on treatments tailored to the individual patient rather than to abstract symptoms.

There has been quite a battle waged during the last century between practitioners of homeopathy and conventional medicine. Through the power and influence of the American Medical Association (AMA), conventional medicine prevailed, and the homeopaths lost influence.

While homeopathy is still practiced today, it has nowhere near the influence it did in the 1900s. (If you are interested in reading about the battle between these warring factions, you should read the book *Copeland's Cure* by Natalie Robins.)

I will use the term "conventional medicine" going forward, and keep in mind that one of the hats I wear as a member of this community of physicians is my operating room cap. Like most conventional physicians, I was trained during medical school and residency for the detection, diagnosis, and treatment of signs and symptoms of disease, without much attention to prevention (and the pharmaceutical companies are eternally grateful). But, as I have mentioned, it is not the only medical hat I wear. Today my focus is prevention combined with healing.

The biggest criticism directed at conventional medicine is its focus on symptoms, which are subjective evidence of disease or physical disturbance. A second criticism commonly leveled at MDs is that they are more adept at writing a prescription—often with side effects that bring new symptoms—to solve a problem, than they are to recommend behavior changes beforehand.

While much of the criticism of modern medicine is warranted, the dedication of nearly all MDs should not be questioned. Physicians want to help; that is why we chose this profession. We really want our patients to get well. It is why we take the Hippocratic Oath, an oath traditionally taken by most physicians affirming their obligation to practice medicine ethically. You may have noticed that I said "most physicians" because, while the oath is considered a rite of passage for practitioners of modern medicine, it is not obligatory and is no longer taken up by all physicians. But that does not mean they are not dedicated and caring doctors. The vast majority of physicians want to provide the best care they are able to offer for their patients. Unfortunately, some are limited by their training, experience, and attitude toward new information.

What Are the Alternatives?

There are other clinical professions that also refer to themselves as "doctors," including the following:

Chiropractic Medicine—This is a health care approach that focuses on the relationship between the body's structure—mainly the spine—and its functioning. Although practitioners may use a variety of treatment approaches, they primarily perform adjustments to the spine or other parts of the body with the goal of correcting alignment problems and supporting the body's natural ability to heal itself.

Naturopathic Medicine—Naturopathic doctors (NDs) are licensed general practitioners specializing in natural medicine. (More on this specialty below.)

Osteopathic Medicine—A doctor of osteopathy (DO) receives training in the body's musculoskeletal system. This training teaches osteopaths to examine, diagnose, and treat the body as a whole rather than treating a single illness or symptom. A doctor of osteopathy takes a more holistic approach to medicine by looking at the body as a complete system instead of placing emphasis on one particular part.

A doctor of osteopathy believes that stress and posture can affect the systems of the body and hinder their proper functions, thus causing disease and illness. Osteopaths also believe that the body has an innate ability to repair and defend itself. In all fifty states, DOs may be trained and licensed to examine patients, prescribe medicine, and perform surgery.

One term you often see connected with alternative therapies is "holistic." Holistic refers to treatments that treat the "whole" body to prevent illness. Holistic practitioners do not wait until a problem arises and then simply cure it, but they consider the body as an interdependent organism to avoid disease. Holistic medicine not only involves the biological body but also includes the psychology, and often the spirituality, of the patient.

All of the types of doctors I discussed above—as well as some of the practitioners below—may be considered holistic. It all depends on their commitment, ideology, and approach.

The Test of Time

Alternative medicine includes a broad range of practices, and many healing therapies are based on ancient Chinese and other Eastern beliefs. Alternative practitioners often point to thousands of years of anecdotal evidence that suggests that certain alternative practices are successful. Today, many people turn to alternative medicine when the traditional medical community cannot help cure them. In some cases, they are using alternative treatments as a first course of action to both cure and prevent illness. There is a growing body of evidence that certain therapies may help improve the quality of life.

Western physicians are slowly coming around and beginning to acknowledge the more established methods of alternative medicine and to recommend alternative therapies for patients they cannot help through conventional medicine. Also, as complementary medicine becomes more acceptable, some medical schools are teaching alternative methods. Fortunately, many physicians now embrace complementary medicine because it creates more options for their patients.

Also, more and more people use alternative medicine to "complement" conventional approaches. This merging of conventional medicine with alternative approaches has given rise to the term "complementary medicine." Recognizing this trend, in 1999 the National Institutes of Health (NIH) established the National Center for Complementary and Alternative Medicine (NCCAM).

The good news is that, as conventional medical practitioners become familiar with alternative approaches, many are incorporating some of the therapies into conventional medicine. This trend is giving rise to integrative medicine (also called functional medicine)—a combination of therapies representing the best of conventional and alternative medicine.

Treatments that incorporate mind, body, and spirit healing are also considered holistic health and can be alternative or complementary.

COMPLEMENTARY/ ALTERNATIVE MEDICINE CATEGORY	EXAMPLES
Alternative medical systems	Acupuncture, Ayurveda, homeopathy, naturopathy, traditional medical systems such as aboriginal, African, Middle Eastern, Native American, Chinese, Tibetan, Central and South American
Mind–body interventions	Art therapy, dance therapy, hypnosis, meditation, mental healing, music therapy, prayer
Biologically-based treatments	Special diets and nutrition therapy, such as the macrobiotic diet, herbal (botanical) therapy, vitamin/mineral therapy, orthomolecular therapy
Manipulative and body-based methods	Chiropractic, massage therapy, osteopathic manipulation
Energy therapies	Biofield therapies, such as Qigong, Reiki, and therapeutic touch; bioelectromagnetic therapies, which involve the unconventional use of electromagnetic fields, such as pulsed fields, magnetic fields, and alternating or direct current fields

SOURCE: *National Center for Complementary and Alternative Medicine (NIH)*

A Word of Caution

While many alternative and complementary therapies may be appealing to you, be careful. Standards are often haphazard if they exist at all. By contrast, conventional medical doctors (MDs) must adhere to well-defined standards and update their knowledge on a regular basis, with Continuing Medical Education courses.

All Natural

Besides my MD background, I also follow a naturopathic philosophy. Naturopaths are holistic and follow the simple concept that our bodies have the inherent ability to maintain and restore health. Naturopathic medicine is based on seven principles of healing. The *Seven Principles of Naturopathic Medicine* are as follows:

1. The Healing Power of Nature (Vis Medicatrix Naturae)

2. First Do No Harm (Primum Non Nocere)

3. Treat the Whole Person

4. Identify and Treat the Cause (Tolle Causam)

5. Prevention Is the Best Cure

6. Physician as Teacher

7. Establish Health and Wellness

I believe a fully integrated—yet simple—plan can lead to the health and wellness we covet and deserve. To achieve optimum health, we must tap our body's inherent desire for wellness. It is not a novel idea, but it is one that has been ignored for too long.

The next section of this book outlines my prescription for optimum health and the payoffs you can expect. I will start with one of life's greatest pleasures: eating.

PART II
The Path to Wellness

C ertainly, regular exercise, a high-quality diet, sensible nutritional supplementation, and improved management of stress all help to ward off major diseases and, in many cases, minimize the need for prescription drugs. But too many of us resist changing habits, and most doctors do not even bother suggesting it. Today's norm is a growing reliance on drugs as the first option.

That's why more than 130 million Americans swallow, inject, inhale, infuse, spray, and apply prescribed medication every month, according to the U.S. Centers for Disease Control and Prevention. In fact, Americans buy much more medicine per person than residents of any other country in the world. We also spend almost as much on drugs as we do to fuel our cars.

It does not have to be this way, not if you follow my four-step prescription starting by adopting a healthier, high-quality diet.

5

Eating Well and Enjoying It

Here is a concept I hope you take away from this book: Food that comes from the ground that is in its most whole form is much better for you than food that is processed or packaged. And food that is grown by small-scale farmers, and especially organic farmers, is, as a rule, more nutritious.

Despite the claims of food manufacturers, studies show that food that has been processed is not nearly as wholesome as food in its original state. Even if the packaging label trumpets "fortified or enriched"—meaning they've tried to add or put back specific nutrients, different from the food's raw and nutritionally dense form—it is not nearly as healthy as nature intended.

Food, in its natural form, provides not only the essential nutrients we need but also other bioactive compounds for health promotion and disease prevention in the proper balance. It is virtually impossible for chemists to duplicate that feat.

But we cannot put all the blame on the food industry. While we all know the importance of a balanced diet, it is common for many people to satisfy their hunger pangs with whatever is near or convenient. This behavior threatens our health; it can also affect our moods and mental abilities.

But even if we recognize that focusing on quality nutritious whole foods yields numerous health benefits and prevents disease, with all the food choices and highly touted diet plans, finding solid and reliable information can be frustrating.

After I began my personal pursuit of optimum wellness, I soon discovered a nutritional approach that made sense and completely altered my outlook on eating. Importantly, it fit perfectly with my quest for high-quality, delicious food that is also satiating. The approach—which has undergone extensive research for over thirty years—is, I believe, the most scientifically substantiated diet program currently available.

This dietary plan is based on a few simple and straight-forward concepts:

▶ There is an ideal human diet that supports and sustains optimum health.

▶ This diet was consumed by thousands of generations of our human ancestors.

▶ Today, in America, the vast majority of our dietary calories come from foods that our ancestors rarely if ever ate . . . and that modern humans are not genetically adapted to eat.

▶ In its current version, this diet closely mimics the nutrition of our evolutionary and genetic heritage.

▶ Consumption of the wrong kinds of foods can lead to cellular imbalances and are a primary cause of many of the chronic diseases seen today.

▶ The result is epidemic levels of cardiovascular disease, cancer, diabetes, obesity, osteoporosis, arthritis, acne, gastrointestinal disease, and more.

Under this diet plan, we should focus on eating lean meats, fish, plenty of seasonal fruits and vegetables, roots, and most nuts. Foods to avoid—or at least limit—include dairy products, grains, salt, refined sugar and processed oils. This is not a raw food diet; foods can and, in many cases, should be cooked.

The diet has a name. It is known as the "Paleolithic Diet," sometimes referred to as the "Stone Age Diet" or the "Cave Man Diet." It is based on what people ate in the Paleolithic or Stone Age era over 10,000 years ago.

The idea first came about in the 1970s and was based largely on research conducted by gastroenterologist Walter L. Voegtlin, who proclaimed that modern humans are best suited genetically for the diet of our Paleolithic ancestors because our genetics have changed little since then. Dr. Voegtlin wrote that humans are carnivorous animals and that the ancestral Paleolithic diet was dominated by fats and protein with only small amounts of carbohydrates. He came to this conclusion based on his own medical treatments of digestive problems, including colitis, Crohn's disease, irritable bowel syndrome, and indigestion.

In 1985, Melvin Konner and S. Boyd Eaton, an associate clinical professor of radiology and an adjunct associate professor of anthropology at Emory University in Atlanta, published a paper on Paleolithic nutrition in the *New England Journal of Medicine*. This helped the dietary concept gain medical recognition and consideration. Other journal articles and books followed—some with twists—adding to the body of evidence that the Paleolithic Diet may help solve many of today's most vexing health problems.

In 2003, the theory gained its greatest mainstream recognition when *The Paleo Diet* by Loren Cordain, PhD, was published. Dr. Cordain is a professor of exercise physiology at Colorado State University in Ft. Collins, Colorado. A self-proclaimed anthropology buff, Cordain wrote the book after twenty years of research on Paleolithic nutrition, habits, lifestyle, and history.

I too believe that the Paleolithic Diet Theory presents a fully integrated, holistic, and comprehensive program and is the best bet to achieve optimum wellness. And there are countless studies to back it up.

If you have never heard of it, your first thoughts might be, "What did they know? They rarely lived past thirty—long before many of our modern diseases existed." If so, consider this: There are still over eighty hunter–gatherer tribes in the world—at least that we know of—and for them, arthritis, diabetes, high blood pressure, heart disease, stroke, many mental diseases, cancer, and other diseases are nonexistent.

Also, our basic genetic makeup has not changed very much. As evolutionary medicine points out, the changes in diet and other lifestyle conditions brought on by the introduction of agriculture and animal husbandry

SEASONAL FOODS

Food is at its most nutritious when it is eaten during its normal growing season. With improved food transport methods, seasonal fruits and vegetables, including organic produce, can originate almost anywhere. However, be aware that standards differ throughout the world. What might be considered organic in another country might not meet the criteria in the U.S. Then there is the cost of transporting food hundreds and sometimes thousands of miles. According to the Organic Consumers Association, the typical American meal consists of an assortment of foods that have traveled an average of 2,000 miles to get from distant farms to our dinner plates.

Ideally, you should eat organic food grown locally and in season. If you are not sure where local organic produce is grown or sold in your area, go to this Web site and enter your ZIP code. You might be surprised. www.localharvest.org.

approximately 10,000 years ago occurred too recently on an evolutionary timescale for natural selection to alter the human genome.

Because it is based on our nutritional needs and is compatible with our genetic code, this diet provides all the critical dietary components, including vitamins, minerals, quality fats, protein, and complex carbohydrates. Many of the proponents of diet say we should derive about 55 to 65 percent of our food energy from animal foods (protein and fats) and 35 to 45 percent from plant foods (complex carbohydrates). This diet achieves that.

The Paleolithic Diet consists of foods that can be hunted—such as meat and seafood—and that can be gathered, such as eggs, fruit, nuts, seeds, vegetables, mushrooms, herbs, and spices. Practitioners are advised to eat only the leanest cuts of meat, free of food additives, preferably wild game meats and grass-fed beef because they contain relatively high levels of omega-3 fats compared with grain-produced domestic meats.

Of course it is not realistic for us to live a hunter–gatherer lifestyle—especially because our landscapes are mostly paved parking lots and roads and very few wide-open plains. To mimic the diet today, proponents have adopted this diet by eating cultivated plants and lean cuts from domesticated animal meat as an alternative to the wild sources of the original pre-agricultural diet.

Foods to Avoid

At this point, you might be rubbing your eyes not believing me when I said earlier that you need to eliminate or minimize dairy-derived products and grains, beans, and potatoes. Because "cavemen" did not have domesticated cows or other milk-producing animals, the dairy part is fairly easy to understand. But why not grains, beans, and potatoes? After all, for many of us these are staples, and the U.S. Department of Agriculture stresses grains in its Food Guide Pyramid. The main reason is that they are inedible—and toxic—when raw. Because Paleolithic humans did not have the capability to cook grains or beans, they would have become deathly ill from the toxins present in these foods, including enzyme blockers and lectins.

Grains contain toxic proteins, including enzyme blockers and lectins—bad-tasting, natural pesticides designed to discourage predators from eating them. These toxic substances ward off a range of species, including bacteria, birds, insects, and mammals—as well as humans. Anthropologic studies of bones and teeth illustrate that populations who added or substituted harvested grains to their Paleo-type diet had shorter life spans, higher rates of childhood mortality, greater incidences of osteoporosis, and various vital nutrient-deficiency diseases, including rickets.

Beans are also full of enzyme blockers (EBs) and lectins, and potatoes contain both plus another type of toxin called glycoalkaloids (GAs). Unlike lectins and enzyme blockers, glycoalkaloids are not destroyed by cooking.

Here is more information about enzyme blockers and lectins:

Enzyme Blockers (EBs)—In addition to grains, beans, and potatoes, these are also found in seeds. As their name implies, they block the enzymes that digest protein (proteases) and are called protease inhibitors. They can affect the stomach protease enzyme pepsin and the small intestine protease enzymes trypsin and chymotrypsin. Some enzyme blockers affect the enzymes that digest starch (amylase) and are called amylase inhibitors.

In human and animal studies, researchers have found that high levels of protease inhibitors promote the pancreas to secrete additional digestive enzymes because the body senses that the level of necessary enzymes has been altered and signals the pancreas to make more. Even a small increase in pancreatic enzyme secretion can add up over time, stressing the pancreas and other organs. When grains, beans, and potatoes are cooked, not all of the enzyme blockers are destroyed.

Lectins—These natural proteins can bypass our normal defenses, wearing away protective mucus from tissues and damaging the small intestine. Lectins can cause cells to act as if they have been stimulated by insulin, while others cause the pancreas to release insulin. Besides being toxic, lectins may also be inflammatory. Although most lectins are destroyed by normal cooking, many are not.

The amount of lectins contained in food depends on the type of plant, how it was processed, and the species. The main foods that may contain toxic lectins include the following:

- Grains—including wheat, quinoa, rice, oats, buckwheat, rye, barley, millet, and corn

- Legumes

- Dairy foods

- The nightshade family—including potatoes, tomatoes, eggplants, and cucumbers

Different lectins are associated with different diseases, including rheumatoid arthritis and adult-onset diabetes, also known as type 2 diabetes. Dairy-based lectins have been linked with juvenile-onset diabetes.

Lectins may also bind to the wall of the gut and may contribute to gastrointestinal diseases such as colitis, Crohn's disease, celiac sprue, peptic ulcers, and irritable bowel syndrome. Because of the damage that lectins do to the lining of the digestive system, it has been suggested that their actions may prevent other proteins from being digested, causing allergic reactions.

Here is another reason to avoid—or minimize—your consumption of potatoes, beans, and grains. After they are cooked, they have a high glycemic index (also known as a sugar spike) because they are loaded with carbohy-drates. Also, after being cooked, they're relatively poor sources of vitamins and other nutrients, especially vitamins A, B-group, folic acid, and C; miner-als; antioxidants; and phytosterols.

Glycemic Index and Blood Sugar

Carbohydrates are one of three macronutrients—protein and fats being the other two—that provide the body with energy. Carbohydrates come in both simple and complex forms. In order for the body to use carbohydrates for energy, food must be digested, absorbed, and metabolized. During metabolism, carbohydrates and oxygen combine producing carbon dioxide, water, and energy. The body uses the energy and water and rids itself of the carbon dioxide.

The glycemic index (GI) is a ranking of foods containing carbohydrates and their effect on blood glucose levels. Because glucose is absorbed into the bloodstream faster than any other carbohydrate, it has been given a value of 100, with other carbohydrates assigned a number relative to glucose. Foods with a low glycemic index release sugar gradually into the bloodstream, producing minimal fluctua-tions in blood glucose. On the other hand, high GI foods are absorbed quickly into the bloodstream, causing an escalation in blood glucose levels. To compen-sate for the rise in blood sugar levels, the body increases insulin production. As a result, high-glycemic-load foods cause us to feel hungry sooner.

Plant-based foods typically exhibit low glycemic indices. Examples of low GI foods include most fruits and vegetables (except potatoes and watermelon), fish, eggs, meat, and nuts. High GI foods include corn, potatoes, watermelon, some white rices, croissants, white bread, candy, chips, and cereals.

Low GI foods decrease the risk of developing diabetes, obesity, and other related syndrome X diseases by placing less stress on the pancreas to produce insulin and by preventing insulin insensitivity. Also, hunger pangs are warded off for longer periods.

Glycemic Load

Glycemic load (GL) takes into account the amount of carbohydrates in a given serving of a food in addition to its glycemic index. Developed by Harvard researchers, it provides a more useful yardstick because it measures not only the glycemic value of each food but also rates them by serving sizes. In general, whole plant foods such as vegetables and fruits have a low glycemic load. Pure whole grains have a lower glycemic index and glycemic load than refined grains or "white flour" products. As a general rule, this means that you can (and should) eat more fruits and vegetables than breads (especially white breads).

Caffeine, Sugar, and Salt

Caffeine

Caffeine is the most popular—and of course, legal—mind-altering drug in the world. It is estimated that 80 percent of the adult population in the United States are regular coffee drinkers.

Caffeine has been the subject of numerous studies investigating whether coffee offers any health benefits. The results are mixed, ranging from "Yes" to "No" with the majority of studies falling in between. While many acknowledge that coffee can provide a boost if consumed in moderation, I say, "Enjoy yourself." There are studies showing it can help you in a myriad of ways.

According to a study published in August 2008 by The American Physiological Society, athletes who ingested caffeine along with carbohydrates had 66 percent more glycogen in their muscles four hours after finishing intense, glycogen-depleting exercise compared to when they consumed carbohydrates alone. (Glycogen is muscle tissue's primary fuel source during exercise.)

Other scientific evidence now suggests that moderate coffee consumption may be associated with reduced risks of certain disease conditions, including Alzheimer's disease, kidney stones, and depression.

Some other studies on coffee include the following:

▶ In 2000, researchers at the Mayo Clinic linked coffee with decreased rates of Parkinson's disease.

▶ In 2004, Harvard researchers reported that coffee significantly reduced the risk of developing type 2 diabetes.

▶ A 2005 study found that coffee helped prevent a type of liver cancer.

One major area of controversy is coffee's effect on heart health. A study published in the *Annals of Internal Medicine* in June 2008 examined the relationship between coffee and mortality. The researchers examined the coffee drinking habits of more than 42,000 men over eighteen years of age, and 86,000 women for twenty-four years. All subjects had no history of cardiovascular disease (CVD) or cancer.

According to lead author Esther Lopez-Garcia of the Harvard School of Public Health, the researchers found that as coffee consumption increased, the overall risk of death—particularly from CVD—decreased. For example, they found that women who drank two to three cups of coffee a day had a 25 percent lower risk of dying from heart disease than non-coffee drinkers.

Lopez-Garcia says this is so because the researchers found that coffee has some beneficial effects on inflammation and endothelial function, which are indicators of the first stages of CVD development.

While there are many studies stating that a moderate number of cups of coffee is perfectly safe, keep in mind that researchers often use a five- or six-ounce cup as a standard. Most people today drink from mugs—which typically equal two cups. Too much caffeine can make you jittery and affect your sleep.

While caffeine contains no calories, many people add sugar and cream. Coffee also increases our desire for sweets, adding even more calories. Also, while coffee has some antioxidant properties, it is no substitute for fruits and vegetables.

Still, as I pointed out, caffeine makes coffee the most popular beverage. If you drink coffee, I suggest limiting consumption to one to two cups a day.

Sugar and Flour

What passes for sugar today contains nothing but calories. It has no vitamins, minerals, or protein—just calories.

White, granular sugar is commonly known as table sugar, but when it is included in foods, it is often called sucrose, glucose, dextrose, fructose, or maltose.

Sugar is one of the most overused foods, and often people do not even know they are eating it. It is been estimated that the average American consumes more than 120 pounds of sugar per year.

What do sugar and white flour have in common? Foods such as pasta and bread are made from white flour with all the essential fatty acids and nutrients removed. When digested—which puts a strain on our gastrointestinal system—flour acts as a simple sugar. As with sugar, it is also added to many foods.

Flour and sugar (as well as brown sugar, which many mistakenly think is better for us) are found in cookies, soft drinks, candies, cakes, and ice cream. They are also added to peanut butter, soups, ketchup, salad dressings, canned fruit and vegetables, and cereals. White flour is often a main ingredient in many fast foods and is added as filler to others, including hot dogs and burgers.

Sugar dependency, or sensitivity, is caused by imbalances in the body and brain chemistry. Our bodies can become used to sugar and begin to crave it. When sugar is removed from our diets completely, we often suffer withdrawal, feeling deprived and occasionally depressed. Sugar cravings can increase over time, and so can one's waistline if he or she gives in to them. With sugar and white flour so abused, it is no wonder our cravings often become a form of dependency.

Systemic Effects of Sugar

Sugar acts more like a drug than a food. For one thing, it quickly passes through the stomach wall, causing blood glucose levels to rise, then fall. As the blood sugar level rises, the pancreas secretes insulin to compensate for the excess blood sugar. As the blood sugar level drops below normal, the result is lethargy, irritability, or depression—commonly known as the "sugar blues."

A strong desire for sweets may very well be due to serotonin, a brain chemical that makes you feel relaxed and less anxious and stressed, and that reduces pain, improves your mood, calms you, and even makes you sleepy. It is suspected that people who crave carbohydrates—including sugar and while flour—have lower serotonin levels, which increases cravings for carbohydrate-rich foods. As serotonin levels increase, research shows that the cravings decrease.

Endorphins may also play a role in our craving for carbohydrates. Endorphins are a group of proteins produced naturally by the body with potent analgesic properties—similar to morphine. (These are the brain chemicals that contribute to the "runner's high" or good feelings during and after exercise). Because sugar affects the release of these powerful chemicals that ease stress and discomfort, endorphin imbalances contribute to obesity and eating disorders. In other words, obese people are probably more sensitive to endorphins' appetite-stimulating effects than are lean people.

Sugar and other carbohydrate foods stimulate the insulin response so that glucose, the end result of sugar and carbohydrate metabolism, is distributed throughout the body from the bloodstream. (Insulin lowers the blood sugar level and triggers hunger.) To process the sugar, the blood sugar level can fluctuate from too high to too low, resulting in a "high" followed by a "low." That's why an unbalanced diet high in simple sugars and low in protein causes a roller-coaster effect on blood sugar levels. To reverse this low, we often seek out snacks, usually carbohydrate-rich foods.

The excessive use of sugar also depletes the body's B-complex vitamins and minerals. This may increase nervous tension, anxiety, negative moods, food cravings, and—in women—PMS symptoms. Too much sugar also intensifies drowsiness by causing the narrowing of the diameter of blood vessels.

For those with an insatiable sweet tooth, artificial sweeteners are not a smart alternative. A recent study by Purdue University researchers found that when rats were fed the artificial sweetener saccharin or sugar, the rats in the saccharin group actually gained more weight than the rats in the sugar group. The researchers concluded that the saccharin-consuming rats came to associate the sweet taste with a reduction of calories, and began to overeat as a consequence.

Do not humans act the same? When we drink an artificially sweetened soft drink, we often accompany it with a snack or we feel hungry sooner. Plus, many artificial sweeteners contain fattening ingredients, including dextrose and maltodextrins, which are known to stimulate fat storage and to elevate insulin.

Salt

Using salt on our foods is a relatively modern development. It certainly did not come from our Paleolithic ancestors. Our bodies only require the small amount of salt that exists naturally in foods. We consume far too much salt and anticipate and crave the taste with certain foods. That is why we "can't eat just one," as the old potato chip slogan trumpeted. It was not the taste of the potato we craved; it was—and is—the salt. The same goes for peanuts, crackers, corn chips, and popcorn dripping with butter (or some high-calorie, artificial concoction resembling butter).

Even though salt is an acquired taste, many people have become so accustomed to it they believe food tastes too bland without its addition. Table salt or common salt is a chemical compound comprised of the minerals sodium and chloride, with the formula NaCl. For many, high salt intake—table salt is roughly 40 percent sodium and 60 percent chloride with a trace of iodine—causes high blood pressure, stroke, and an accumulation of fluid, called edema.

But even if you do not add salt to your meals, most packaged foods, including soups, pickles, canned goods (including vegetables), beans, peanut butter, bread, macaroni and cheese, ketchup, mustard and relish, processed meats, and dressings—have added salt. Fast foods, including hamburgers, hot dogs, french fries, pizza, and tacos, are loaded with salt.

We do need salt. However, if you eat fruits, vegetables, nuts, and seeds on a regular basis, you are probably getting enough of this important mineral.

There is a big difference between natural and table salt. Natural sodium in fruits and vegetables is combined with other organic molecules. Unlike natural sodium, which is absorbed slowly by our bodies, table salt is unbuffered and enters quickly through the stomach lining.

When this surplus salt enters the bloodstream, the body is forced to store the salt between the cells until filtered by the kidneys. To protect themselves, cells release water into the intercellular fluid to dilute the excess salt. As the cells give up their water, they lose elasticity and shrink, causing a chemical imbalance in the cells through a loss of potassium.

This can become a vicious cycle. Low potassium levels cause more sodium to penetrate the cell walls; when the sodium level of the cell rises, water then enters to dilute it, causing the cell to become swollen. It is estimated that one ounce of salt causes the body to hold six pounds of excess fluid.

In the worst-case scenario, the continuous disruption of the cell's fluid balance can, in time, calcify, scar, and even destroy muscles, valves, and arteries. Eventually, this can result in serious medical conditions such as congestive heart failure and other life-threatening conditions.

Our Need for Quality Protein

In addition to providing energy, our bodies need protein for growth, cellular maintenance, regeneration and repair, and other essential body functions such as hormone and enzyme production. More importantly, proteins are vital for fluid balance within cells and for maintenance of normal blood pressure.

Amino acids are the building blocks of protein. Long chains of amino acids, called polypeptides, make up the multicomponent, large complexes of protein. There are twenty different forms of amino acids that the human body uses.

Eleven amino acids are considered nonessential. This means the body is able to synthesize them. The remaining nine amino acids are classified as essential—which means the body is unable to synthesize them. These must come from our diet.

When we eat protein, our bodies use the essential amino acids from foods to synthesize some of the nonessential amino acids. Because we are constantly turning over protein in our bodies, the replenishment of lost amino acids is one of the most important aspects of protein intake. That is why we need to eat quality protein—to ensure that our bodies have the right balance of amino acids to replace the lost amino acids. This ensures optimum maintenance and growth and overall health.

Animal proteins such as eggs, meat, and fish are considered high-quality, or complete, proteins because they provide sufficient amounts of the essential amino acids. Plant proteins—including grains, corn, nuts, vegetables, and fruits—are incomplete proteins because they lack at least one essential amino acid, or they lack a proper balance of amino acids.

Some Facts About Fat

In today's world, fats deliver much of the flavor and help determine the texture of many foods. For many of us, our taste buds have become accustomed to high-fat foods, and therefore we may not find low- or normal-fat food very satisfying. As a result, many people indulge in higher-fat foods more often than they should.

Here are few important definitions:

Saturated fat—This type of fat can cause atherosclerosis or clogged arteries. Foods high in saturated fat are composed of animal products, including meat, poultry, butter, whole milk, and tropical oils, such as coconut, palm, and palm kernel. Eating too much saturated fat increases the risk of cardiovascular disease.

Polyunsaturated fat—Polyunsaturated fats can help reduce high blood cholesterol levels. These are usually liquid or soft at room temperature and include safflower, sunflower, corn, sesame, and soybean oils, as well as certain types of fish.

Monounsaturated fat—Monounsaturated fats can also help decrease high blood cholesterol levels when they are part of a reduced-fat diet. They are usually liquid at room temperature and include olive oil, canola oil, peanut oil, avocados, and nuts.

Trans fat—Trans fats occur when fat is hydrogenated, chemically converting it from a liquid vegetable state to a more solid whipped or stick state. This process creates compounds called partially hydrogenated fats, or trans fats, which studies have shown to raise levels of the bad cholesterol (LDL) while lowering good cholesterol (HDL). Small amounts of trans fat can occur naturally in dairy products and other foods of animal origin, but most of the trans fat in the American diet is found in margarine, commercial baked goods, and fried foods.

Essential fatty acids (EFAs)—The essential building blocks of dietary fats are fatty acids. Once fats are consumed, they are broken down into fatty acids, which are used for energy, growth, development, and important cellular components. Our bodies can produce most of the fatty acids we need, but certain essential fatty acids cannot be generated by the body and must be obtained in our diets. The two main essential fatty acids are omega-6 and omega-3.

The ratio of omega-6 to omega-3 that we consume in our daily diet is important and can have significant health effects. Most of us consume too much omega-6 and too little omega-3 because the typical American diet is overloaded with omega-6 fats and contains insufficient omega-3 fats. The current ratio of omega-6 to omega-3 fatty acids in the U.S. diet is about 10:1, whereas in our ancestors' hunter-gatherer diets, it was closer to 2:1. This dietary imbalance in fatty acids (excessive omega-6 and insufficient omega-3) is a fundamental underlying cause of many chronic diseases in our society, including cardiovascular disease,

DRINKING WATER ADVICE

Water is essential for all life to exist, as it makes up more than 70 percent of most living things, including the human body. While a human can survive more than a week without food, a person will die within a few days without an adequate water supply.

Water serves as a solvent for nutrients and delivers them to cells while also helping the body eliminate waste products. Water lubricates joints and acts as a shock absorber inside the eyes and spinal cord. Water also helps the body maintain a constant temperature, similar to a thermostat.

Water is the recommended beverage on the Paleo Diet. I recommend you drink plenty of water to aid in your body's ability to metabolize stored body fat efficiently. A dehydrated body tends to retain fat. Even though people trying to lose weight often avoid adding to their water weight, the truth is that drinking plenty of water is absolutely necessary for your body to decrease stored fat.

It is recommended that adults drink eight to ten 8-ounce glasses of water a day. While that may sound daunting, remember that many foods and beverages contain water, which can make up part of this daily intake. For example, fresh and cooked vegetables and fruits contain up to 90 percent water, and meats contain at least 50 percent.

Bottled waters are usually quite expensive, and there is the added concern of plastic bottles clogging up landfills. A good filtering system attached to a kitchen tap plus an unbreakable water bottle, for mobility, are excellent investments.

many cancers, inflammatory disorders, and many psychological disturbances. Omega-3s are particularly important for brain and vision development in infants and may affect learning, memory, and stress levels throughout life.

A completely fat-free diet is not healthy. In addition to loss of the essential omega-3 and -6 fats, reduction or elimination of dietary fat can cause insufficient absorption of fat-soluble vitamins. It also will not help with weight management if you do what most people do—replace fatty foods with fat-free, high-calorie options. This is one of the key fallacies of foods advertised as "fat free."

Researchers from the Tufts University School of Nutrition Science and Policy say the smartest thing to do is reduce your intake of both saturated and trans fats. These nutrition experts say the key to eating fat, losing weight, and staying healthy is to focus on eating monounsaturated fats. Monounsaturated fats are found in olive oil, fish, and some vegetables. These fats may lower your cholesterol, and, when used in moderation, should not interfere with healthy weight management.

At the same time, avoid saturated fats found in fatty meats, dairy products, and coconut and palm oils, and trans fats found in many processed foods, including margarine and chips. These can raise your cholesterol levels and increase your risk of heart disease.

Oleic acid is the major monounsaturated fat in our diets and is found in meats, nuts, avocados, dark chocolate, and olive oil. As pointed out in a *Mayo Clinic Proceedings* review article from January 2004, entitled "Becoming a 21st-Century Hunter-Gatherer," although some of these foods were not part of the ancient ancestral diet, they can improve the cardiovascular risk profile when substituted for sugar, starches, trans-fats, and saturated fats that are prevalent in the modern diet. Studies suggest that replacing saturated fat with monounsaturated fat would result in a 30 percent reduction in cardiovascular risk, or three times the risk reduction achieved by replacing saturated fat with carbohydrates.

Why Organic Foods Are Better

Organically grown food is free from exposure to harmful chemicals, including herbicides and pesticides, but it is actually more than that. Organic agriculture involves the health of the soil and of the ecosystems where crops

SAFE FISH TO EAT

In 2004, a joint draft fish advisory from the U.S. Food and Drug Administration and the U.S. EPA added tuna—America's second-most popular seafood after shrimp—to its list of mercury-containing fish that should be restricted in the diets of pregnant women and young children. A separate new study found unhealthy pollutants in far higher concentrations in farmed salmon vs. salmon caught in the wild.

Because mercury is stored in our bodies, as it is in fish, women planning to have children should also avoid high-mercury fish well before they become pregnant. According to a study by the Centers for Disease Control, 16 percent of American women of childbearing age have levels of mercury in their blood high enough to indicate increased chance of harm to their fetuses.

The FDA and EPA advise that young children, pregnant women, nursing mothers, and women of childbearing age not eat more than two or three meals, or 12 ounces total, of fish or shellfish a week. They should limit high-mercury fish to one serving per week.

and livestock are raised. A healthy growing environment significantly benefits crops and, by extension, the health of those consuming them. In addition, organic practices are better over time because they are efficient in their use of resources and do not damage the environment.

In addition to avoiding added hormones, antibiotics, or other drugs, there are a number of nutritional benefits from meat, eggs, and dairy products from pasture-raised over feedlot-raised animals. For example, meat from grass-fed cattle is lower in total fat. If the meat is very lean, it can have one-third as much fat as a similar cut from a grain-fed animal. Grass-fed beef can be as lean and have the same amount of fat as a skinless chicken breast.

Because meat from grass-fed animals is leaner, it is also lower in calories. Fat has 9 calories per gram, compared with only 4 calories per gram for protein and carbohydrates. The greater the fat content, the greater the number of calories. For example, a 6-ounce steak from a grass-fed steer can have 100 fewer calories than a 6-ounce steak from a grain-fed steer. Also, meat from grass-fed animals has two to four times more omega-3 fatty acids than meat from grain-fed animals. Meat from organically grown animals is also richer in antioxidants, including vitamins E, beta-carotene, and vitamin C.

When chickens are housed indoors and deprived of greens, their eggs and meat are lower in omega-3s. Eggs from pastured, free-range hens can contain as much as ten times more omega-3s than eggs from factory hens.

Meat and dairy products from grass-fed animals are the richest known source of a health-promoting fat called conjugated linoleic acid, or CLA. When

FISH TO AVOID

The following are fish eating guidelines from the EPA and the USDA:

High mercury: Atlantic halibut, king mackerel, oysters (Gulf Coast), pike, sea bass, shark, swordfish, tilefish (golden snapper), tuna (steaks and canned albacore)

High persistent organic pollutants (POPs): Farmed salmon. Limit to once a month if pregnant/nursing. Check TheGreenGuide.com periodically for updates on POPs in other farmed fish.

FISH TO EAT

Moderate mercury: Alaskan halibut, black cod, blue (Gulf Coast) crab, cod, Dungeness crab, Eastern oysters, mahi mahi, blue mussels, pollack, and tuna (canned light). (Children and pregnant or nursing women are advised to eat no more than one from this list, once a month.)

Low mercury: Anchovies, Arctic char, crawfish, Pacific flounder, herring, king crab, sand dabs, scallops, Pacific sole, tilapia, wild Alaska and Pacific salmon, farmed catfish, clams, striped bass, and sturgeon. (Children and pregnant or nursing women can safely eat items from this list two to three times a week.)

Environmentalists point out that low-mercury but overfished or destructively harvested species include Atlantic cod, Atlantic flounder, Atlantic sole, Chilean sea bass, monkfish, orange roughy, shrimp, and snapper.

livestock are raised strictly on a fresh pasture-fed diet, their products contain three to five times more CLA than products from animals fed conventional diets. This may be important because CLA may be one of our most potent defenses against cancer. In a study appearing in the journal *Cancer,* researchers found that, in laboratory animals, a very small percentage of CLA greatly reduced tumor growth. It is theorized this may also be true for humans.

However, if you want to continue to consume dairy products, it is important to remember that low fat is still fattening; for example, when you drink 2 percent milk, while it is 2 percent fat by weight, it is 33 percent fat by calories.

The 80/20 Rule

I realize that some of my advice, such as the recommendation to avoid or limit consumption of dairy products, grains, salt, and refined sugar, may be hard for people to accept. However, limiting one's consumption of these foods, even to a small extent, can still yield great benefits. Consider adopting the strategy I prescribe for my patients at The Wellness Center—what I call my 80/20 rule. The 80/20 rule recommends that people try to achieve a healthy diet and lifestyle 80 percent of the time; the other 20 percent—perhaps during the holidays or on a weekend day—they can indulge themselves, but of course not go overboard. With my patients, I have always maintained a realistic and pragmatic attitude. If I can help someone whose diet is 20/80 move closer to a healthy diet—perhaps a respectable 50/50 diet—that at least is a start on the path to wellness for that person.

Let Food Be Thy Medicine

Hippocrates said it centuries ago, and the food industry is finally discovering ways to fulfill his edict with what is known as functional or super foods. Functional or super foods provide significantly higher levels of nutrients than the other typical foods many of us eat every day.

The demand for functional food is being driven by a growing public awareness and understanding of the link between diet and disease. One category of functional food that has grown by leaps and bounds in the last few years is the so-called functional beverage—usually juices from exotic fruits such as acai, gac, goji, wolfberry, mangosteen, etc., supported by other fruit or vegetable juices. These beverages may also have certain specific nutrients or extracts—such as amino acids, essential fatty acids, or minerals—added in as well. Most of these beverage products are designed to function as foods; they provide good taste, energy, and basic nutrition while offering the purported enhanced health benefits.

Most of these beverage products boast very high levels of antioxidant components to protect against chronic diseases such as heart disease, dementia, cancer, and arthritis. Many others focus their benefits on improving immune function and reducing inflammation levels in the body.

We have all heard the recommendation to eat a wide variety of colored fruits and vegetables each day, particularly ones with deep colors like dark red, orange, and yellow. It is plant nutrients, or so-called phytonutrients, that give plants their color. For example, carrots get their orange from a group of fat-soluble compounds called carotenoids. Beta-carotene, lycopene, and lutein are carotenoids that have been studied extensively for their antioxidant properties.

Superfruits from tropical or exotic locations around the world often contain unique phytonutrients that confer added health benefits when consumed by humans. Fruits originating in the wild have evolved to be reasonably robust and resistant to natural environmental stresses, diseases, insects, and other predators. Many of the fruits and berries grown on so-called factory farms in the U.S. and around the world have been bred over the last 50 years to have the sweetest taste, to be uniform in size, or to have the ability to withstand shipment. That type of growing process does not necessarily produce fruits with the best or highest amounts of phytonutrients, like we see in superfruits.

One of the most important functions of color in plants, or specifically, plant pigments, is not simply to please our eyes but to protect the plant from the sun's harmful rays. The sun is required for the plant to conduct photosynthesis. At the same time, the UV rays from the sun can be harmful to the plant in that they promote free radicals. These unstable oxygen molecules produced during plant metabolism are kept in check by these plant phytochemicals.

When we consume the plant and the phytonutrients that go along with it, these same protective effects are conferred upon us. Adequate levels of antioxidants neutralize oxidative stress, counteract adverse effects of aging, support cardiovascular and immune function, and promote overall health and wellness.

A wealth of scientific studies has demonstrated that the natural pigments that give fruits and vegetables their vibrant hues offer remarkable health benefits. Powerful antioxidants, these phytonutrients are linked with health benefits that include protection from cancer, cardiovascular disease, dementia, diabetes, and stroke, just to name a few.

A test that is commonly used to measure the antioxidant capability of foods is called ORAC. This test measures the ability of foods to subdue harmful free radicals that can damage our bodies. (See box.)

WHAT ORAC REPRESENTS

As I mentioned earlier in the book, antioxidants provide health benefits by subduing free radicals, which play a role in the development of many age-related diseases. The antioxidant value of a food can be estimated using a measure called oxygen radical absorbance capacity, or ORAC. Foods with a higher ORAC value possess a higher ability to quench dangerous oxygen free radicals in the test tube. Scientists have found that boosting your daily intake of foods with high ORAC values increases the body's plasma and tissue antioxidant protection, guarding your body's tissues against the onslaught of free radicals that can lead to decay and disease.

USDA scientists recommend obtaining 3,000 to 5,000 ORAC units each day—far more than what most individuals consume. Increasing consumption of high ORAC-value fruits and vegetables provides a simple yet powerful method of increasing the body's defenses against disease-provoking free radicals.

POPULAR SUPERFRUITS *(In alphabetical order)*

- Acai
- Acerola
- Aronia
- Bilberry
- Caja
- Camu-camu
- Cranberry
- Elderberry
- Goji
- Mangosteen
- Pomegranate

Superfruit Advice

If you decide to go the functional, superfruit beverage route, allow me to make a few suggestions. Make sure the drink is made primarily from whole fruit purees and not simply freeze-dried, concentrated, or processed fruit extracts. Also, verify that the main or most beneficial ingredients are offered in meaningful concentrations so as to provide the stated benefits.

My Diet Prescription

There is a growing body of evidence that diets containing moderate amounts of beneficial fat and protein in addition to foods consisting primarily of low-gly-cemic-load carbohydrates—non-starchy vegetables and fruits—in conjunction with daily exercise, is the most effective way to achieve and maintain ideal body weight and prevent cardiovascular disease. Because this was the eating pattern and lifestyle of prehistoric humans, you should consider following the Paleo Diet.

If you do, you should avoid or at least limit the following (remember the 80/20 rule):

- ▶ Grains—including bread, pasta, noodles
- ▶ Beans—including string beans, kidney beans, lentils, peanuts, snow peas, and peas
- ▶ Potatoes
- ▶ Dairy products
- ▶ Sugar
- ▶ Salt

Instead, eat the following:

- ▶ Pasture-fed, lean red meat and free-range chicken and fish
- ▶ Eggs
- ▶ Fruit—especially berries such as blueberries, raspberries, and strawberries; includes superfruits such as acai, pomegranate, and acerola

▸ Vegetables—especially root vegetables such as carrots, turnips, parsnips, and rutabagas—but limit potatoes or sweet potatoes

▸ Nuts—including walnuts, Brazil nuts, macadamias, and almonds (minimize peanuts [a bean] and cashews)

Notes About Eggs

Try to eat eggs from organic, free-range chickens because they have a far superior balance of omega-6s to omega-3s than grain-fed poultry. They also have lower cholesterol. Also, poach or hard boil the eggs. These methods of cooking eliminate the fat and calories used in frying.

How many eggs? Clinical tests conducted at the Medical College of Pennsylvania in 1992 found that people on a low-fat diet who ate twelve eggs a week did not increase their serum cholesterol level. Frankly, for many people, I believe that is too many eggs.

When you hear concern expressed about eggs, much of it centers on the egg yolks rather than the white portion. As Dr. Cordain points out in a supplemental report to The Paleo Diet, egg whites are a complex healthy mixture of forty proteins. However, egg yolks are also of nutritional value because they are one of the densest sources of the important B vitamin and biotin, while raw egg whites contain a glycoprotein called avidin that can bind with biotin and prevent its absorption.

Here is what I suggest: while studies show little or no harm in egg consumption from free-range, organically grown chickens, if your doctor has told you to be careful about your lipid profile, limit your consumption of whole eggs to about four per week.

Getting Started

Following this diet requires a little planning on a meal-to-meal, daily, and weekly basis. If you decide to get started, follow my 80/20 rule (adhere to the diet guidelines 80 percent of the time).

Some changes require minimal behavioral modification. For example, when selecting carbohydrates, instead of drinking orange juice, eat the orange, or, when eating out, substitute starches like potato or rice with an extra serving of vegetables.

Eating healthy foods is only one change we must make if we want vibrant health and wellness. In today's environment, it may be more important than ever to incorporate nutritional supplements in our wellness plan to ensure we are receiving all the nutrients our bodies need.

6

Supplement Your Health

In the last chapter, I offered my nutritional guidelines and the recommendation to adopt the principles of the Paleolithic Diet. As I mentioned, this approach to eating is not a simply a weight loss plan as the term diet might imply, but instead, a health-promoting lifestyle based on eating fresh fruits and vegetables, lean protein, and unsaturated fats.

By adopting this dietary approach, I indicated that the essential nutrients and other bioactive compounds for health promotion and disease prevention could be obtained in proper balance. If this is true, then why do I recommend taking nutritional supplements?

The reality is that most people do not adhere to a health-promoting diet the majority of the time. With busy and often stressful lives, it can be difficult to eat properly. Even if you are conscientious, you face challenges. In some parts of the country, particularly during the colder months, it can be difficult to obtain fresh fruits and vegetables. Instead, the only produce available has probably been picked before it was ripe and flown to regions far away, so that by the time the produce is eaten it may have limited nutritional value.

To help counteract this, nutritional supplements can help. As the term supplementation implies, nutritional supplements are intended to cover the gaps in diet—not make up for an unhealthy lifestyle. If it is not possible to consume fresh fruits and vegetables—which are loaded with vitamins, minerals, antioxidants, and other phytochemicals—it makes sense to obtain these nutrients from supplements as a form of nutritional insurance policy.

In the last twenty-five years, our understanding of nutrition has grown tremendously. For example, recent studies revealed a positive relationship between higher levels of vitamin D intake and lower rates of colon cancer in adults. Based on this compelling finding, the researchers recommend that adults obtain 1,000 IUs of vitamin D on daily basis—a level much higher than the current recommended dietary allowance (RDA) of 400 IUs. To obtain this level of vitamin D through food alone would be difficult. However, by augmenting a healthy diet with a vitamin D supplement, this goal is much more attainable.

Nutritional Supplement Pyramid

During consultations with patients at The Wellness Center, many sought my advice regarding the selection and use of nutritional supplements. Even the most educated and nutrition-savvy patients found it difficult to determine which supplements were best suited to meet their nutritional needs.

To help guide my patients, I developed a tool called the Nutritional Supplement Pyramid. This tool was designed based on the well-known Food Guide Pyramid to ensure a logical approach to nutritional supplementation.

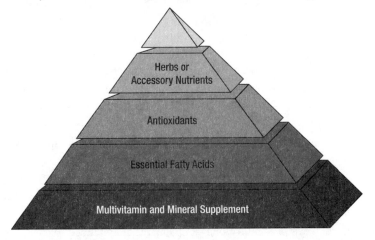

The Nutritional Supplement Pyramid is based on four recommendations to establish a solid nutritional program.

▶ First, take a good quality multivitamin and mineral supplement to cover gaps in your diet.

▶ Second, add a good source of essential fatty acids (EFAs), especially omega-3 fatty acids.

▶ Third, take extra antioxidants for free-radical protection.

▶ Fourth, once you have met your requirements for these basic nutrients, add any additional herbs or other nutrients to meet your specific health and wellness goals.

This section of the book is not intended to provide extensive information regarding vitamins and minerals. A number of well-written books have already been published on the subject. In particular, I recommend that my patients refer to *The Encyclopedia of Nutritional Supplements,* an excellent guide written by Michael T. Murray, ND. His companion book, *Encyclopedia of Natural Medicine,* is also an excellent resource.

Instead, my intention is to provide you with the necessary guidelines to use when selecting vitamin and mineral supplements. Here is more information about each of these recommendations.

1. Multivitamin and Mineral Supplements

In 2002, two Harvard researchers published a report in the *Journal of the American Medical Association* indicating that all Americans should take a daily multivitamin. The recommendation was based on research demonstrating that daily use of a multivitamin may help prevent a number of chronic diseases, including heart disease, some cancers, and osteoporosis.

You can be sure research will continue to evaluate the merits of supplementation with specific vitamins and minerals in the prevention and treatment of chronic disease. Meanwhile, the majority of Americans should take a multivitamin and mineral on a daily basis to cover gaps in their diet. Essentially, taking a good quality multi is like taking out an inexpensive insurance policy to protect one of your most important assets—your health.

As with many things in life, not all supplements are created equal. When evaluating a product, the following should be taken into consideration:

Optimal Dosing. Many multivitamin and mineral supplements are touted as providing 100 percent of the RDA for a broad range of nutrients. For example, One-A-Day Women's is formulated with 100% of the RDA for both vitamin C and vitamin E. Surprisingly, when I question my patients, most assume that the RDA for vitamin C is 500 mgs and for vitamin E is 400 IUs. In actuality, the RDA for vitamin C is only 60 mgs and for vitamin E just 30 IUs!

If you are obtaining just 100 percent of the RDA from your supplement products, you might not be getting enough of certain nutrients. This distinction is important because the RDA often reflects the minimum requirement needed to prevent deficiency diseases. These allowances do not take into consideration that higher levels of certain nutrients may be beneficial in the prevention of chronic degenerative diseases such as heart disease, cancer, and stroke. For this reason, the RDA is viewed as being deficient, particularly as it relates to key antioxidants such as vitamin E and vitamin C. Instead, optimal daily intakes (ODIs) have been established by industry leaders and better reflect requirements based on recent findings from research and longitudinal studies.

Morning/Evening Dosing. The advantage of a one-a-day multivitamin is that it is simple and convenient to take. However, the ideal way to take a multivitamin is in a morning and evening formulation. The use of daytime and nighttime dosing, or chronotherapy, provides the right nutrients at the right time of day. Divided doses also ensure optimal absorption of the water-soluble vitamins including vitamin C and the B-complex.

Natural Vitamins. Not all vitamins are available in the natural form. But wherever possible, the natural form should be selected, as research has demonstrated that this form is more readily absorbed than its synthetic counterpart. In the case of vitamin E, the natural form is indicated as "D," as in d-alpha-tocopherol, whereas in the synthetic form, it is referred to as "D-L," as in dl-alpha-tocopheryl acetate. Manufacturers often use the synthetic form because it is less expensive.

Vitamin Families. Vitamin E does not refer to just one compound but to a family of eight compounds: four tocopherols and four tocotrienols. The B-complex also refers to a family of eight vitamins, including niacin, riboflavin, and folate. In nature, these vitamin families tend to appear together, creating synergistic, beneficial effects. When isolated in a supplement form, their benefits are less well understood. When supplementing with vitamin E or the B-complex, I recommend that the entire vitamin family be taken to optimize the health benefits.

Chelated Minerals. Our bodies have a difficult time absorbing minerals in supplement form. The use of chelation—a technology that attaches an amino acid to minerals—facilitates mineral absorption.

No Iron. A multivitamin and mineral supplement should not contain iron. Supplemental iron should only be taken by individuals who are iron deficient. Also, for better absorption, iron should be taken separately from other nutrients.

No Artificial Ingredients or Herbals. Nutritional supplements should not contain any preservatives or colorants, which can cause allergic reactions in some individuals. Examples include FD&C yellow #6 and FD&C blue #2 lake—common ingredients in less-expensive supermarket and drug store brands. A multivitamin should not contain any herbs, as these botanicals should typically be taken in a separate formulation.

(For a list of vitamins and minerals and the roles they play in the body, see Appendix C on page 150.)

2. Essential Fatty Acids

After covering gaps in your diet by taking a high-quality multivitamin and mineral supplement, the next step is to take an essential fatty acid (EFA) supplement. It would be best to obtain the important omega-3 fatty acids that our bodies require from foods. However, for some individuals who dislike seafood, this can be problematic because it would be necessary to eat cold-water fatty fish, such as salmon or mackerel, on a frequent basis. Also, because of concerns about ocean pollution and farm-raised fish having lower levels of omega-3s, supplementation is a wise alternative.

Like vitamins and minerals, EFAs are essential nutrients that our bodies require and, if not obtained from diet, need to be supplemented. Because most people do not eat enough fruits, vegetables, nuts, and seeds and consume too many processed packaged foods, their diets lack in essential fatty acids.

EFAs perform a number of vital functions in the body but are particularly important at the cellular level because they are a fundamental component of the membranes of all cells. An adequate supply of EFAs in the diet is also essential for healthy-looking skin because skin cells turn over very rapidly.

The two essential fatty acids—alpha-linolenic acid (an omega-3 fatty acid) and linoleic acid (an omega-6 fatty acid)—are very important to the health of the body. In addition to alpha-linolenic acid, the omega-3 family of essential fatty acids includes eicosapentaenoic acid (EPA) and docosahexaenoic acid (DHA). As omega-3 fats, both EPA and DHA promote the development of favorable prostaglandins—hormone-like compounds that play a role in inflammation, blood pressure, kidney function, blood clotting, and platelet aggregation. Although our bodies are able to convert alpha-linolenic acid to EPA and DHA, our ability to form these important compounds is limited. This is why these two fats are considered conditionally essential.

If you would like to learn more about the role of fats in health and disease, I recommend the book *Fats that Heal, Fats that Kill*. The book is written by Udo Erasmus, who is considered to be one of the foremost experts in the field of fatty acid nutrition.

An excellent source of EFAs is flaxseed oil, one of the world's richest sources of omega-3 fatty acids. Flaxseeds should be expeller-pressed for their oil at low temperatures without exposure to damaging light, oxygen, and reactive metals. Whether encapsulated or in liquid form, flaxseed oil should be packaged in bottles that do not expose the delicate oil to damaging light.

Certain types of fish and fish oil contain high levels of EPA and DHA. Supplementing the diet with these high-quality fish oils leads to the production of health-promoting prostaglandins. In particular, EPA and DHA are well-documented to benefit cardiovascular health by lowering cholesterol, making the blood less sticky, and decreasing the incidence of abnormal heart rhythms. This is an important consideration given that cardiovascular disease is the number-one killer for both men and women in this country.

Compared with flaxseed oil, the quality and types of fish oil supplements vary widely. While fish oil supplements can be purchased cheaply on the Internet, it is often difficult to know where these products were sourced and ultimately their quality. The best quality fish oil supplements are manufactured by companies like Ocean Nutrition (Nova Scotia, Canada), who own or control the entire production process, from managing the fish stock to extracting the oil from the fish.

3. Antioxidants

Earlier in this book, I explained how antioxidants play a protective role against the development of heart disease, cancer, and other chronic degenerative diseases by quenching free radicals. Antioxidants are also believed to slow down the aging process by reducing the body's oxidative load. In other words, antioxidants slow down the internal "rusting" of our bodies as we age.

Although vitamins and minerals play a role in growth, maintenance, metabolism, and many other bodily functions, a number of these micronutrients also function as antioxidants. Vitamins C and E are good examples. Both vitamins, which are commonly formulated in a multivitamin and mineral, support overall health and wellness while providing excellent antioxidant protective benefits.

If a typical multivitamin provides nutrients that have antioxidant benefits, why is it necessary to supplement with additional antioxidants? One reason is that some of the most potent antioxidants like green tea and grape seed extract are not found in a typical multinutrient formula. Another reason is that supplementing with a broader range of antioxidant nutrients protects a wider number of systems in the body. That is because certain antioxidants operate in specific parts of the body.

The carotenoid lutein, which is found in yellow and dark green leafy vegetables, provides a good example. Lutein is highly concentrated in the macula region of the retina and is deposited in the epidermal and dermal layers of the skin. Lutein filters high-energy blue light, which is very damaging to the macula of the eye and skin. By absorbing blue light and reducing oxidative damage in the macula, lutein protects against age-related macular degeneration (ARMD), the most common cause of blindness in Americans aged 60 and older.

Based on extensive data, it appears that a combination of antioxidants provide greater antioxidant protection than any single antioxidant. Therefore, in addition to recommending that individuals consume a diet rich in plant foods, especially fruits and vegetables, research suggests using a combination of antioxidant nutrients rather than high dosages of any single antioxidant. Mixtures of antioxidant nutrients appear to work together harmoniously to produce the phenomena of synergy. In other words, 1 + 1 = 3.

Some key antioxidants to consider adding to your daily supplement regimen include the following:

Vitamin A and Carotenoids—A number of my patients have voiced concern about taking vitamin A supplements. Because this vitamin is stored in the liver and other tissues, it can be toxic if taken in high doses over time. While this is a valid concern, it is important to understand the source of vitamin A, as this will determine your intake of this nutrient.

Vitamin A in its pure form is often referred to as retinol, palmitate, or preformed A. Good sources of vitamin A are found in products of animal origin such as liver, kidney, egg yolks, butter, and whole milk. Even if you do not consume these foods, your vitamin A intake might be higher than you think. Federal law mandates that nonfat and low-fat dairy products be fortified with vitamin A. Additionally, many functional foods and meal replacement products are fortified with vitamins and minerals, including vitamin A.

OVERCOMING DIETARY DEFICIENCIES CAN IMPROVE BEHAVIOR

In a blind trial conducted in England in 2003, researchers found that changing prison inmates' diets cut violent behavior by 35 percent. In the study, one group of prisoners was given a multivitamin mineral and fatty acid supplement while another group was given a placebo. The study was carried out at Aylesbury Young Offenders Institute by the research charity Natural Justice led by Bernard Gesch, a senior research scientist at Oxford University's physiology department.

The study began again in earnest in 2008. In the study, volunteers from three young offenders institutions housing male prisoners aged 16 to 21 began taking nutritional supplements on top of their normal choice of food to ensure they receive the necessary vitamins, minerals, and essential fatty acids to meet daily guidelines. The results will be compared with a control group under double-blind conditions. Researchers will monitor how levels of nutrients affect a range of behaviors, including violence, drug-related offences, and incidents of self-harm.

Some members of a group of fat-soluble plant compounds called carotenes or carotenoids can also convert into vitamin A and, as such, are termed provitamin A. However, not all carotenes convert as readily into vitamin A. Because beta-carotene converts the most readily, this form is often used in nutritional supplements. However, some carotenes, such as lycopene, zeaxanthin, and lutein, do not have any provitamin A activity (do not convert into vitamin A). Instead, they exert potent antioxidant protective benefits.

The recommended dietary allowance (RDA) for vitamin A is 5,000 international units (IUs). A supplement that contains 5,000 IUs of vitamin A from a retinol source would satisfy 100 percent of the RDA requirement. However, a supplement that contains 15,000 IUs of vitamin A from a carotenoid source (e.g., beta-carotene) is not providing three times more vitamin A than the RDA. This is because it takes six to twelve times more carotenoids to convert into one international unit of retinol.

Importantly, the body only converts carotenoids into vitamin A as needed. As vitamin A stores in the body are fulfilled, the conversion process is decreased. For this reason, carotenoid intake can be considerably higher than 5,000 IUs and still present no safety or toxicity issues.

Vitamin C—A water-soluble vitamin whose primary role is to protect the watery (aqueous) part of cells. Vitamin C is incorporated into an enzyme that helps stabilize collagen, promotes the healing of wounds, and protects against blood clotting and bruising.

Vitamin E—An important fat-soluble vitamin that prevents the oxidation of fats. Vitamin E actually refers to a family of eight compounds: four tocopherols and four tocotrienols. Some members, such as alpha-tocopherol, are the most potent in terms of vitamin E activity. Other members, like delta-tocotrienol, have more potent antioxidant, cholesterol-lowering, and anticancer effects. To obtain the full benefits, it is best to take a supplement that provides all members of the vitamin E family—similar to how this vitamin is found naturally in foods.

Selenium—A trace mineral that inhibits the oxidation of fats and protects vitamin E. Selenium is incorporated into glutathione peroxidase, an enzyme that has peroxidase activity and protects our bodies from oxidative damage.

Alpha-Lipoic Acid—A versatile antioxidant that functions in either water-soluble or fat-soluble environments. Alpha-lipoic acid also regenerates other antioxidants.

Grape Seed Extract—A powerful antioxidant with excellent bioavailability that strengthens collagen. Grape seed helps to cross-link collagen fibers, preventing collagen destruction.

Green Tea Extract—Contains protective compounds called polyphenols that have antioxidant activity and may provide protection against skin cancer.

Ginkgo Biloba Extract—Powerful antioxidant herb known for increasing circulation and has antiaging properties.

Milk Thistle—A powerful antioxidant that contains potent liver-protecting substances. The active compound silymarin also stimulates the production of new liver cells.

4. Botanicals and Accessory Nutrients

Once the body's requirement for the above basic nutrients has been met, targeted supplements can be added to address specific health issues. These typically include herbal supplements but can also include enzymes, amino acids, and others.

As the name implies, accessory nutrients are not essential in the human diet but, when taken, can be useful for solving a variety of health problems. Examples include glucosamine sulfate, which is used by many for mild to moderate symptoms associated with osteoarthritis. Here are some other examples:

▶ **Asian Ginseng** (Chinese and Korean) to increase energy, endurance, and libido.

▶ **Bilberry** to increase microcirculation by stimulating new capillary formation, strengthening capillary walls, and increasing overall health of the circulatory system.

▶ **Echinacea** to prevent and treat the common cold and upper respiratory tract infections.

▶ **Ginger** to treat nausea, motion sickness, and vomiting and increase appetite.

▶ **Ginkgo biloba** to enhance memory.

▶ **St. John's Wort** or **Sam-E** to reduce anxiety and mild depression.

▶ **Saw Palmetto** to counteract the symptoms associated with an enlarged prostate.

▶ **Valerian** to relieve anxiety and nervous irritability. Also used as a sedative and sleep aid that is non-habit-forming.

A Precautionary Note

You may have heard that you should ask your doctor whether a supplement interferes with any prescription medicine you are taking. This is a wise thing to do, but it actually brings up another important issue. What has received little publicity or attention until recently is how many prescription drugs and over-the-counter medications disturb the body's ability to absorb nutrients. As a result, when you use some medications, not only are you increasing the load of possibly toxic chemicals in your body, you might be starving it of essential nutrients, which could exacerbate the health problem for which you are taking the drug or cause you to develop new disease symptoms. This could lengthen the period of recovery.

7

Exercise and Wellness

Think about it. When we were young, many of us played stickball, dodgeball, tag, hopscotch, and red light/green light, and we flew kites and jumped rope for hours on end. We were in motion all day long and usually only took breaks for meals or naps.

As for adults today? Unfortunately, at some point, many of us just stopped moving. Did our bodies tell us to make this behavioral change? No. Many of us have settled for more sedentary activities to relax and pass the time—like watching television with a remote control from a recliner.

Studies show that nearly 30 percent of Americans engage in no physical activity, and an additional 60 percent engage in less than 30 minutes of activity per day. Here's a sad statistic: the number of deaths in the U.S. related to sedentary living or obesity is approximately a half million per year.

Our ancient ancestors moved and exercised their muscles every day. If they didn't, they starved.

The Value of Exercise

Our bodies are designed for movement. Our muscles, joints, ligaments, and cartilage allow us to walk, run, jump, reach, and throw things. Without a doubt, the old adage is true: "If you don't use it, you lose it."

To achieve and maintain a high quality of health, physical activity is vital to wellness. There is abundant scientific research documenting the association between physical activity, health, longevity, and an improved quality of life. Physical activity may affect quality of life in several ways: it can be used to improve self-image, self-esteem, and physical wellness, and it can promote optimal health.

Consider this:

> ► It might seem contradictory, but a lack of energy is largely a result of inactivity. Endurance exercises such as walking, swimming, jogging, biking, and rowing improve stamina and energy. After just a few weeks in a walking program, most people find they have more energy for activities such as gardening and traveling.

> ► As stated in a previous chapter, researchers have found a link between regular physical activity and improved immune function.

> ► There is ample evidence that exercise provides many benefits to help people look and feel younger.

> ► Exercise triggers the release of endorphins in our bodies—our natural tranquilizers and pain relievers. As a result, exercise reduces stress.

In addition to the obvious benefits of exercise—decreased weight and increased strength and energy, for example—it can reduce the risk of developing chronic ailments and ease the symptoms of others. For one thing, workouts are important for the health of our digestive systems. Exercise improves digestion, promotes the assimilation of food, and facilitates elimination of waste from the body, thereby stimulating the lymphatic system, which is partly responsible for the removal of toxins from the body.

Exercise also can help to reduce blood viscosity. By thinning the blood, exercise helps to keep blood flowing and also maintains the integrity of our blood vessels. Wide-open blood vessels allow the blood to flow easier, meaning improved circulation all the way to our capillaries. Furthermore, exercise strengthens the heart, lowers cholesterol levels and triglyceride counts, and—if done regularly and with moderation—decreases resting high blood pressure.

MOOD ELEVATOR

In addition to its physical health benefits, regular exercise helps elevate one's mood. A number of studies have shown that exercise can lift a person's spirits, and there is even evidence that physical activity can aid in treating clinical depression. This study, appearing in the *Journal of Sports Medicine and Physical Fitness* in December 2001, focused on depressed mood, rather than clinical depression.

In the study, researchers found that different types and intensities of exercise have varying effects on individuals' moods. The researchers studied eighty young men and women who agreed to mood tests before and after an hour-long aerobics class.

The investigators determined that fifty-two volunteers were in depressed moods before the exercise, while twenty-eight were not. After exercise, the depressed-mood group was significantly more likely to report a reduction in anger, fatigue, and tension, as well as increased vigor.

Other studies have suggested that, for some patients, regular activity may be a better depression treatment than psychotherapy or medication. Exactly why is unclear, but studies show that exercise can positively influence certain mood-related hormones.

Exercise also improves the condition of other vital organs, muscles, bones, joints, and tissue. A recent report from the Harvard Center for Cancer Prevention concluded that following a low-fat, high-fiber diet and increasing exercise could reduce half of all cancer risks. Physical activity is believed to reduce cancer risk by influencing levels of hormones and other growth factors, strengthening the immune system, and decreasing body fat.

One of the main goals of exercise is to improve our body composition—the relative proportion of fat-free mass to fat mass in the body. Fat-free mass is composed of muscle, bone, organs, and water, whereas fat is the underlying adipose tissue. Excessive fat is a good predictor of health problems because it is associated with cardiovascular disease, high cholesterol, and high blood pressure. Higher proportions of fat-free mass indicate an increase in muscle and thus an increased ability to adapt to everyday stress.

Getting physical is beneficial—and necessary—for everyone, and can be started during any stage of life. One goal of Healthy People 2010, a set of national health objectives established by the U.S. Department of Health and Human Services, is to increase the number of people participating in daily physical activity. The activities can vary, ranging from a structured exercise program to team sports, including bowling. Even simple tasks that we like to farm out to others—such as housework, walking a pet, mowing and raking the yard, or walking (instead of driving) around town when running errands.

I personally enjoy a variety of sports and physical activities. Workouts at the gym, personal training, snow skiing, walking, hiking, and yoga are some of my favorites. I try to achieve a mixture of indoor and outdoor activities, so I

EXERCISE MAY REVERSE PREDIABETES IN ADULTS

In an article appearing in the March 26, 2003, issue of *Diabetes Care*, researchers found that inactive adults who add a few hours of exercise each week may cut their risk of developing a prediabetic condition known as insulin resistance syndrome, even if they do not lose weight. Because the population is eating more and exercising less, increasing numbers of adults and children are developing the syndrome, which results when a person loses the ability to use insulin effectively. The syndrome can develop into type 2 diabetes and increase the risk of heart disease if left untreated.

To investigate whether physical activity influences the risk of insulin resistance syndrome, researchers followed eighteen sedentary men and women for six months. Participants exercised by walking for thirty minutes between three and seven days a week, and they were told not to change their diets or body weights. At the end of the study, researchers examined insulin sensitivity and levels of blood fats such as cholesterol. They found that exercise alone increased insulin sensitivity.

According to researchers, even modest amounts of exercise can improve indicators of glucose and fat metabolism among inactive, middle-aged adults—a group that is particularly at risk for developing type 2 diabetes—even without a loss of abdominal fat or weight.

rarely get bored. I also try to use a variety of muscle groups and capabilities to maintain my weight, muscle tone, and balance.

As I emphasize to all my patients, it is important to vary one's exercise routine to maximize the benefit. The important thing is to find a way to incorporate exercise you will enjoy so you will look forward to (and not dread) lacing up your sneakers or walking shoes.

Our goals should include the following:

Muscular Strength—This refers to the maximum amount of force a muscle can exert with a single effort. Strong muscles are important not just for sports, but for everyday tasks such as carrying groceries, doing yard work, and climbing stairs. Muscular strength can also help to keep the body in proper alignment, prevent back and leg pain, and provide support for good posture.

Muscular Endurance—This is the ability of a muscle or group of muscles to perform repetitive contractions over time. Endurance is important, even for everyday activities. Along with strength, it helps maintain good posture and prevent back and leg pain. It can also help in dealing with everyday stress.

There are three kinds of exercise I stress to my patients:

▶ Resistance exercise

▶ Cardiovascular activities

▶ Flexibility movements

Resistance Exercise—This includes lifting weights, performing isometrics, and doing other resistance-type exercises. The goal with resistance exercise is to build and maintain muscle mass. As we age, we lose muscle mass. At approximately thirty years of age, we have built up the maximum amount of skeletal muscle in our bodies we are ever going to have. From that point on, we lose muscle cells; either they die or become damaged. If we do not do something to maintain our muscle mass, we will lose it—both in functionality and strength.

The good news is that you can overcome the loss of muscle mass—and it is possible to maintain or increase your strength at any age. In a well-known study at a nursing home, after embarking on some lightweight training and resistance exercises, people aged ninety and above who were initially bedridden were able to get out of bed, and others were able to discard their walkers. Just building up their muscle mass to a small degree helped tremendously with their ability to move and perform basic life functions. In this regard, maintaining our muscle mass and building up strength is vital for healthy aging.

Just remember, you need to carry out weight or resistance training, especially after age thirty, throughout your life. When it comes to muscle, you either use it or lose it. Just as important, if you lose muscle mass, the percentage of body fat goes up, and the percentage of lean body mass goes down.

Another important point is that building up your skeletal muscles is a great way of burning calories and thereby maintaining body weight. This is why weight lifters can consume a tremendous number of calories. Because muscle burns more calories than fat does, the more muscle you have in relation to fat, the higher your basal metabolic rate. The bottom line is that strength training is important for almost any fitness goal, whether you want to lose fat, gain muscle, or simply improve your conditioning.

Cardiovascular Fitness—This refers to the ability of the body to perform prolonged, large-muscle, dynamic exercise at moderate to high levels of intensity. This ability is dependent on the ability of the heart and lungs to deliver oxygen to the working muscles. As fitness levels improve, the body becomes more efficient and can better withstand the challenges of everyday stress.

Cardiovascular exercise, or cardio, is necessary to maintain your cardiovascular system, including all of your blood vessels and your heart. You can accomplish this and reap the benefits by walking or running—whatever revs up the heart. Normally the body maintains its cardiac output by pumping about five liters of blood per minute through the heart. When we exercise, we increase this output to approximately twenty-five to thirty liters per minute, a five- to sixfold increase. The cardiovascular system has a tremendous capacity to increase its output, but to maintain this level of fitness, you need to exercise the heart on a regular basis.

Flexibility—This refers to exercise that affects a joint or group of joints. Flexibility becomes more important as people age and their joints stiffen up, preventing them from doing everyday tasks. If you do not move your joints, they get stiff over time and lose functionality, including range of motion.

EXERCISE ON THE CHEAP

You do not have to buy expensive equipment, hire a personal trainer, or join a gym to enjoy fitness. Because results are all that matters, use what you have: a pair of sneakers, a jump rope, even sandbags and paint cans for weight training. The American Council on Exercise recommends walking, jogging, dancing, and bike riding as cost-effective means to conserve gasoline while losing weight. Household chores also are useful to increase metabolism and energy level.

Here are simple ways to cut costs and stay in shape (according to the American Council on Exercise):

- Walk or bike to work. Each burns calories, saves money on transportation, and helps the environment.
- Find a park with a fitness course. Follow the directions on the obstacles for a pleasant exercise session in the fresh air.
- Volunteer to clean up a park in your neighborhood. Vigorous chores like yard work are great calorie burners, and this would be a great way to improve the neighborhood, meet neighbors, and make new friends.
- Buy a jump rope. Jump rope for fifteen to twenty minutes a day, three days a week.
- Use video on demand. You can access workout videos cheaper than purchasing a DVD.
- Choose activities that get you moving. Go to the park, walk the dog, play catch, and plan trips with family and friends that involve activities such as biking, paddleboating, hiking, swimming, skiing, or just walking to a museum.
- Park away from your destination. Stop driving around looking for a close parking space. Park in the spot that is farthest from the mall or grocery store, and get some exercise.
- Take the stairs. Climbing the steps at work or other buildings burns a lot of calories and really revs up the heart.

Good range of motion allows the body to maintain good posture. Stretching is therefore an important habit to start, as well as continue, as we age. Yoga is a good example of a type of stretching exercise. (Also, if you play a sport or take part in a running or walking program, you should stretch beforehand.)

The important point is that we have to do all three types of exercise—resistance, cardiovascular, and flexibility—to stay healthy as we age.

Anaerobic and Aerobic Exercise

Exercise is also classified as anaerobic or aerobic, depending on the energy pathways that are used during exercise. Most everyone is familiar with aerobic exercise; not everyone is as familiar with anaerobic exercise. There is a difference between the two, and training techniques can enhance both of them.

Typically, anaerobic-type exercises are high intensity and last only a few seconds up to a few minutes. They are commonly used by athletes (especially bodybuilders) to help build power and muscle mass.

Aerobic exercise is less intense but lasts for longer periods than anaerobic exercise. Aerobic exercise is primarily used during endurance-type athletic events. Examples include walking, running, dancing, and boxing. The good news is that moderate exercise can be just as beneficial as vigorous exercise.

CHORES BURN CALORIES

You do not have to adopt an extra workout regimen when so many of your household chores burn plenty of calories.

Examples include (according to the American Council for Fitness and Nutrition) the following:

- Mowing the lawn (30 minutes) = 150 calories burned
- Gardening (30 to 45 minutes) = 150 calories burned
- Raking leaves (30 minutes) = 150 calories burned
- Vacuuming (30 minutes) = 100 calories burned
- Washing windows (15 minutes) = 50 calories burned
- Sweeping (15 minutes) = 50 calories burned

The American College of Sports Medicine recommends performing an aerobic activity four to five times weekly for thirty minutes at a moderate to vigorous intensity. Women have been known to obtain even more benefits from exercise. Those who exercise regularly have lower rates of breast cancer as well as other cancers, such as colon cancer.

Exercise May Slow Aging

The American College of Sports Medicine, the CDC, the Surgeon General, and other health-promoting associations have all formally recommended physical activity for everyone. Their goal is to make everyone aware of the health benefits from regular physical activity while also indicating the amount and intensity necessary for optimal health.

A study appearing in the *Journal of Sports Medicine and Physical Fitness* in 2000 found, after conducting an analysis of thirty-seven studies, including 720 adults aged forty-six to ninety, that middle-aged and elderly individuals may be able to slow some of the effects of aging on the cardiovascular system by using exercise. In those studies, people participating in thirty minutes or more of exercise three times a week, and who achieved at least 80 percent of VO_2 max—the maximum oxygen consumption, which is a measure of the ability to transport and use oxygen during exercise—were able to slow the decline in cardiovascular health that accompanies aging.

The researchers discovered that individuals who exercised at this level for more than fifteen weeks showed no significant benefits over those who exercised for fewer than fifteen weeks, suggesting that improvements can be made in less than four months and then maintained after that point. Researchers found no difference in fitness between those who walked and jogged and people who cycled. To get the desired results, the researchers recommended that people—with their doctor's approval—need to participate in strenuous exercise for at least a half-hour three times a week.

Exercise Functional Payoffs

There are numerous benefits associated with regular participation in an aerobic exercise program. I have already touched on these, but they bear repeating and expansion.

Aerobic exercise improves cardiovascular and respiratory functioning—including lowered blood pressure and increased efficiency of the heart—with a commensurate reduction in coronary artery disease risk. Improvements in cardiovascular and respiratory systems include greater efficiency by exercising muscles to use oxygen and lowering resting and exercise heart rates. Also, stamina increases and fatigue is reduced. This can mean improved diabetes management and reduced bone-mineral loss. Although exercise in general can increase strength, muscular endurance, and flexibility, cardiovascular exercise has the most dramatic effect on the body because it engages large muscle groups in an aerobic manner.

Exercise in Disease Prevention

In addition to having an effect on heart disease, studies show that exercise also can have a direct effect on preventing several types of cancer—including breast, prostate, and lung cancer—and other causes of premature death. Research also shows that aerobic exercise can reduce obesity and osteoporosis. In addition, risk of high blood pressure, blood clots, and stroke can also be reduced with regular physical activity.

Physical activity can reduce the risk of colon cancer by as much as 50 percent, and it can reduce the risk of developing type 2 diabetes and coronary artery disease by similar amounts. Over age fifty, as many as one in four women and one in eight men are at risk for development of osteoporosis. The risk of osteoporosis is reduced through regular physical activity in all age groups—children, adolescents, and adults.

Even more important, several of these factors are interrelated. For example, when an individual lowers his or her high blood pressure, the risk for heart disease, stroke, and kidney disease is also reduced. Another example is that exercise favorably alters blood lipid profiles, including total cholesterol (TC, the complete count of all cholesterol in the blood), high-density lipoprotein cholesterol (HDL-C, the good cholesterol), low-density lipoprotein cholesterol (LDL-C, the bad cholesterol), and triglycerides (TG, storage form of energy), which reduces the risk of plaque buildup in coronary arteries, a factor that may lead to coronary artery disease.

Getting Started

It is easy to get confused about exercise—how many minutes a day should we spend working out, for how long, and at what exertion level? Conflicting facts and opinions abound, but the bottom line is this: regular exercise—including a walking program—is good for you, whether the outcome measurement is blood pressure, diabetes, cardiovascular disease, overcoming stiff joints, or improving mental health. Walking does not cost you anything, and you can do it at a place and time of your choosing—even right now!

My Exercise Prescription

As I tell my patients at The Wellness Center, adequate physical activity is dependent on having a well-rounded program that encompasses all aspects of improving health and preventing disease. This includes cardiovascular fitness, muscular strength and endurance, flexibility, posture, and maintenance of body composition.

For most people, getting started is the most challenging part of regular exercise. Having a goal can help you stay motivated. Your goal may be to lose weight, lower your total cholesterol, or improve your body tone. We

DIET HAS GREATER IMPACT THAN EXERCISE ON WEIGHT GAIN AND LOSS

While exercise is a great weapon to burn calories and ward off diseases, it does not always mean you will lose weight. According to a study appearing in the medical journal *Obesity* in September 2008, it is more important for people—even those who exercise—to change their diets if a goal is weight loss.

In the study led by Loyola University Health System in Chicago, researchers compared African-American women in metropolitan Chicago with women in rural Nigeria. The average weight of the Chicago women was 184 pounds, the Nigerian women, 127 pounds—even though their levels of physical activity were comparable. The big difference in weight, the researchers concluded, was related to their diets; they discovered that while the Nigerian diet was high in fiber and carbohydrates and low in fat and animal protein, the Chicago diet was 40 to 45 percent fat and high in processed foods.

each have to determine the motivation that works best for us to make fitness a lifelong habit. Importantly, making a commitment to lead a more active lifestyle certainly does not translate to a life of harsh discipline. It always helps to have fun. Pick activities that you enjoy. Do not make exercise just another obligation. Try to rediscover the joy of moving. Develop a support network. Find exercise partners. Reward yourself for your progress.

Begin by assessing your goals, your interests, and how ready you are to begin an exercise routine. Prepare yourself for exercise by obtaining the right shoes, clothing, and equipment. Have your fitness level assessed by a fitness professional, such as a personal trainer, physical therapist, or physician. Fitness testing is commonly offered in gyms and health clubs. Or, you can simply begin by asking your friends who exercise regularly for advice or guidance in getting started.

A good example of an exercise program I recommend includes three stages. The first stage is a warmup, during which one performs light calisthenics to activate and warm the muscles, immediately followed by stretching, which helps to maintain flexibility. The second stage is the conditioning stage, which consists of cardiovascular work to enhance the function of the heart and lungs and a resistance-training regimen to strengthen and tone major muscle groups, such as the quadriceps, hamstrings, chest, biceps, triceps, back, and abdominals. The final stage consists of a cooldown, or reduction in heart rate to resting levels, as well as stretching again, because the greatest modification in flexibility comes from postexercise stretching.

Continuity of physical activity is important to maintain a healthy lifestyle. In addition, it is important to follow an exercise regimen that will start slow and gradually increase as fitness level and exercise tolerance increases. The key is to complete at least thirty minutes of activity most days of the week in the form of activities that one enjoys, such as walking, jogging, swimming, aerobic dance, biking, skateboarding, or participating in a sport. This will enable an individual to reach the goals of Healthy People 2010, which include improving the quality of life through fitness with the adoption and maintenance of regular exercise and physical activity programs.

One of the best payoffs from exercise is stress reduction, which is a key component of wellness, as you will read in the next chapter.

8

Stress Management

When I began medical school, I was simply not prepared for the frenzy of activity, demands on my time, or the sky-high expectations of the medical faculty. At first I thought I was lacking in dedication, brainpower, and endurance. At times, the thought even occurred to me that I might not be suited for a career in medicine. But after comparing notes with my fellow student sufferers, I realized we were all in the same boat. Unfortunately, we all thought our boats were sinking, and we did not have the skills to cope.

The constant stream of classes, labs, clerkships, criticism during rounds, and workload from professors piled up and overwhelmed us. The cumulative effect was a level of stress that caused all of us to question whether we were there to learn to help people with medical problems or to be guinea pigs for lab studies of body and mental meltdowns. What I am describing is called stress, which all of us experience daily and most do not handle too well.

Our physical response to stress is something rooted in our genetic code and physiology. When attacked, prehistoric humans needed to react quickly to escape harm; their bodies reacted by releasing substances such as cortisol and adrenaline, which made their pulse and breathing quicken. Blood and oxygen rushed to their muscles and brain, and their digestive system slowed. Blood sugar rose to boost their energy reserve, and their muscles tensed in preparation for movement. This visceral fight-or-flight response was the body's way of mustering all resources to ensure optimal performance. Once the danger passed, early man calmed down and resumed his normal activities.

Psychological stress refers to the emotional and physiological reactions that occur when a person faces a situation above his or her normal coping ability. The reaction and effects from stress vary by individual and by gender; what is stressful for one person is not necessarily stressful for another. Common stressful situations include financial worries, relationship problems, time stress, pressure at work or school, death of a loved one, and health worries and problems.

The biological concept of stress can be broadly defined as challenge— physical and psychological—requiring us to adapt. In fact, our response to stress can sometimes be of benefit, and we can be strengthened by the experience. The benefits cease when the stress is unyielding, we react or cope poorly, or we do not seek relief.

Worry Affects Our Health

It is common for everyone to worry from time to time, but persistent worry can harm the health of your brain. In 2006, an alarming study by the British insurance company Bupa found that people are worrying a great deal more than they did five years ago. Among the most common worries, health topped the list—especially worries about heart disease and cancer. I find it ironic that the primary worries people have about their health—particularly heart disease and cancer—are two largely preventable and treatable conditions.

There is additional interesting data from the study. The researchers found that stress-related medical problems are also becoming more common, including anxiety-induced insomnia. More than a third of those surveyed reported frequently being unable to sleep. Also, over two-thirds of the study participants admitted to being chronically worried, and more than one in five considered taking medication for it.

The Bupa study emphasizes an important point: Emotions—including worry and fearfulness—can have a significant impact on your health, both positive and negative. While it is normal to worry on occasion, and although being fearful is an ingrained trait of survival, too much of either can have serious health consequences—research shows that worry can increase the risk of developing Alzheimer's disease.

Studies show that a positive mental attitude—which includes dealing with fears and worries—can help you cope with or even avoid many health concerns, including these:

▶ Cancer

▶ Heart disease

▶ Arthritis

▶ Autoimmune diseases

▶ Menopause symptoms

▶ Recovery from surgery

I survived medical school and then found that working as a medical professional was every bit as harried and stressful. As much as I love being a doctor and helping people, I realized I had to develop a strategy for dealing with stress. Fortunately, I did.

When I set out on my wellness quest, I discovered and studied under the guidance of Jon Kabat-Zinn, the founder and former executive director of the Center for Mindfulness in Medicine, Health Care, and Society at the University of Massachusetts Medical School. He is also the founder (1979) and former director of its renowned Stress Reduction Clinic and is a professor of medicine emeritus at the University of Massachusetts Medical School.

Jon Kabat-Zinn is credited with developing the program of Mindfulness-Based Stress Reduction (MBSR). First introduced in 1979, MBSR is now offered in over 200 medical centers, hospitals, and clinics around the world. More than 17,000 people have completed the MBSR program. I am proud and feel privileged to be one of their early students.

This is a slight oversimplification, but MBSR combines mindfulness meditation and yoga. MBSR is an eight-week intensive training in mindfulness meditation, based on ancient healing practices. I found that mindfulness practice provided me with a greater awareness of the unity of mind and body as well as the ways that unconscious thoughts, feelings, and behaviors can undermine emotional, physical, and spiritual health.

Dr. Kabat-Zinn teaches that the mind and our resulting thoughts and reactions are key factors in stress and stress-related disorders. Meditation has been shown to affect many autonomic physiological processes positively, such as lowering blood pressure and helping us to react rationally and not emotionally, when appropriate. In fact, a study appearing in the March 2008 issue of the *American Journal of Hypertension* finds that the regular practice of Transcendental Meditation may have the potential to reduce both systolic and diastolic blood pressure.

In addition to mindfulness practices, MBSR uses martial arts to counteract disuse atrophy from our culture's largely sedentary lifestyle, especially for those with pain and chronic illnesses. The program also combines meditation and yoga so the advantages of both can be experienced simultaneously.

What Is Stress?

When we experience stress, the body responds immediately. The brain begins to produce higher levels of hormones, like adrenaline, cortisol, and cortisone. It also halts the production of chemicals, like dopamine and growth hormone. These latter hormones, especially dopamine, are necessary for mood balance.

Other effects of stress on the body include a rapid heart rate and breathing, increased blood flow to the muscles and brain, and decreased blood flow to the digestive tract. Perspiration and muscle tension also result from stress.

Everyone experiences stress, but if neglected or if it becomes chronic, it can cause our health to deteriorate. Learning to cope with and reduce stress is the key to a happier, more balanced life.

If ignored, the effects of stress on the body can become cumulative. The longer and the more frequently we get stressed, the more likely we will start having health problems.

Symptoms due to stress may include anxiety, fatigue, insomnia, sleep disturbances, stomach problems, sweating, racing heart, rapid breathing, shortness of breath, and irritability.

I have seen problems with patients recovering from surgery due to excessive stress. Many chronic health problems are associated with sudden or long-term stress and include the following:

▶ Alcohol abuse

▶ Asthma

▶ Chronic fatigue syndrome (CFS)

▶ Drug abuse

▶ Erectile dysfunction and infertility

▶ Fibromyalgia

▶ Headaches

▶ Heart disease

▶ High blood pressure

▶ Immune system dysfunction

▶ Indigestion

▶ Irritable bowel syndrome (IBS)

▶ Mood disorders, including anxiety and depression

▶ Rheumatoid arthritis

▶ Skin disorders

▶ Slow and impaired wound healing

▶ Stroke

▶ Weight gain and weight loss

Stress has also been documented to cause an accumulation of fat around the abdomen. Several research studies have focused on how the hormone cortisol tends to stimulate fat storage around the stomach.

Stress can also lead people to engage in negative behaviors that actually worsen their stress and their health. Often, people cope with stress by smoking, overeating, or abusing alcohol or drugs. While these strategies may seem to relieve stress temporarily, they also contribute to overall poor health and risk factors for disease that may lead to heart disease, high blood pressure, and stroke. In other words, we exchange our outward stress for internal and self-generated stress.

Chronic stress can lead to insomnia, panic attacks, and anxiety. Long-term effects of stress can alter a person's ability to fully participate and enjoy his or her life.

Eating Away Your Stress

Stress causes some people to avoid eating. This can be a mistake. There are a number of foods that provide the body with nutrients that can help counteract the effects of stress. Here are a few examples: Vegetables are rich in a number of nutrients that can ease the symptoms of stress. Collards, kale, and turnip greens provide significant amounts of riboflavin and some of the other B vitamins that are important to maintaining a balanced emotional and mental state.

Fruits can also help to lower stress. Tomatoes are one of the best examples. Tomatoes have abundant amounts of vitamin A and antioxidants that help maintain the body's immune system. A healthy immune system helps prevent impaired function of our nervous system, which can occur if the stress is constant and lasts for prolonged period of time.

Other fruits that can help alleviate stress are apples, pomegranates, and pineapple because all contain histidine, an amino acid that helps reduce stress. Bananas can also help. They provide potassium, which is shown to have a positive impact on mood and coping ability. Fruits such as oranges that contain a healthy dose of vitamin C are among foods that can help mitigate stress.

Flaxseed is a good source of fiber and alpha-linolenic acid (an omega-3 fatty acid) and is a major source of lignans that reportedly influence hormone function. One study found that adding 30 grams of freshly ground flaxseed to the diets of postmenopausal women on a daily basis reduced the blood-pressure-elevating effect of mental stress and reduced stress-related changes in fibrinogen—a blood component associated with increased risk of heart disease. However, the flaxseed had no significant effect on blood levels of an adrenal stress hormone.

Stress-reducing foods are also found in meat, poultry, and seafood. Fish and poultry are good sources of niacinamide (vitamin B3) and can help to regulate mood. Various meats and fish supply vitamin B12, which provides energy and aids in the maintenance of mental clarity.

Foods that lower stress also typically contain several other essential vitamins and minerals that help maintain multiple body systems. This means that while you combat stress with your diet, you are also providing nourishment for all parts of your body.

Exercise Away Your Stress

As mentioned in the last chapter, there is considerable evidence that regular physical activity can help reduce stress. It can also help with related maladies including mild to moderate depression and anxiety. There is a cascading effect; exercising can improve sleep, boost mood, and enhance the overall sense of well-being—reducing stress even more.

Consider this: studies have found that regular exercisers score higher on measures of psychological well-being and perceived stress, and that people who improve their exercise habits develop changes in their mental attitudes that are associated with better resistance to stress.

In one study, researchers found that a single session of aerobic exercise reduced anxiety, which carried over to a later experience that was psychologically stressful. But even a minimum amount of exercise helps. Aerobic fitness studies have found that people with higher fitness levels are not significantly different from those with lower fitness in resisting the effects of stress. One study gave mentally stressful tests and found no differences between aerobically fit and minimally fit women in physical or psychological measures of stress reaction.

Age and Stress

Aging may be more related to reactions to stress and the absence of disease rather than to a person's chronological age, according to researchers in the fields of neurobiology and psychoneuroendocrinology. Presenting their findings at the 114th Annual Convention of the American Psychological Association (APA) in August 2006, they concluded that healthy aging is more likely if stress can be moderated along with adopting an active, healthy lifestyle.

In one presentation at the conference, Elissa S. Epel, PhD, of the University of California, San Francisco, said that some diseases begin when tissue-building growth hormones (anabolic), including testosterone, estrogen, and thyroid hormone, start to drop off when catabolic hormones such as cortisol, glucagon, and adrenaline increase. When catabolic hormones become too active, they can actually weaken the body. Epel's research found that one of these stress-reacting hormones, cortisol, becomes increasingly reactive when responding to stress-related challenges as we age.

Epel said her research found an imbalance between the anabolic and catabolic hormones that is likely to be responsible for many of the psychiatric and medical diseases associated with aging. She said that, according to a model of neuroendocrine aging, subtle yet chronic changes in hormonal patterns can exert pathological effects on health over time.

It is also known, according to Epel in a press release from UCSF, that chronically elevated cortisol reduces lean body mass and bone density and shifts fat distributions that can precede the onset of many age-related diseases like osteoporosis, metabolic syndrome, Alzheimer's disease, and major depression. But, she added, certain behavioral factors like lifestyle and exercise can modify some of these hormonal effects that seem to accelerate aging.

Compared to healthy older adults under 100 years of age, healthy centenarians, said Epel, tend to show slower insulin and glucose rates

SUPPLEMENTS THAT MAY COMBAT STRESS

Combating stress is one of the most common reasons given for taking supplements, even though human research on the effects of supplements on stress is sparse. With this in mind, consider adding the following supplements to your diet (under the guidance of your health care provider, of course):

Studies of athletes have shown that vitamin C supplementation (1,000 to 1,500 mg per day) can reduce stress hormone levels after intense exercise.

In the field of anesthesiology, surgical patients given 2,000 mg per day of vitamin C during the week before and after surgery demonstrated a more rapid return to normal levels of several stress-related hormones compared with patients not given vitamin C.

In one study, young adults took 3,000 mg per day of vitamin C for two weeks and then were given a psychological stress test involving public speaking and oral math problems to solve. Those taking vitamin C rated themselves less stressed, scored better on an anxiety questionnaire, and had smaller elevations of blood pressure. They also returned to lower levels of an adrenal stress hormone more quickly following the stress test than did a placebo group.

Several studies have evaluated a daily supplement of vitamin B1, vitamin B2, vitamin B3, vitamin B6, vitamin B12, vitamin C, pantothenic acid, folic acid, biotin, calcium, magnesium, and zinc for combating stress. Researchers report that subjects involved in preliminary trials of this combination of nutrients have improved concentration and mood with less fatigue. More research is needed.

when fasting, have higher or similar thyroid hormones, and have similar cortisol and growth hormone levels.

Even though older adults may be exposed to multiple chronic stressors—more health problems and fewer social connections—they do not always experience greater daily stress. The authors believe that the healthy centenarians are using coping techniques such as finding meaning in activities and strengthening meaningful social ties to help moderate chronic stress.

Epel said studies on aging have discovered that centenarians report using three coping strategies to deal with their health problems: acceptance, not worrying, and taking things one day at a time. Those older adults who do not employ these types of strategies may become more vulnerable to stress over time, she added.

Many of the neuroendocrine changes that occur with aging are not inevitable, writes Epel, and are demonstrated by healthy centenarians. Certain age-related changes can be modified with physical activity, sufficient sleep, and good coping techniques. Epel noted, that when chronic stress, inactivity, and added body weight take hold, the neuroendocrine system may become imbalanced. This imbalance between the anabolic and catabolic hormones now appears to be the most common profile of aging and may be a valuable marker for biological aging.

Meditation—An Antidote to Stress

Yoga and meditation are long-term interests of mine. Importantly, modern medical practitioners have begun to appreciate the ability of these simple modalities to reduce stress and enhance overall well-being. Research confirms this, and studies show that meditation may even have the potential to heal. In one study appearing in the June 12, 2006, issue of the *Archives of Internal Medicine,* researchers reported their findings on the effects of Transcendental Meditation (TM) on components of metabolic syndrome. Metabolic syndrome is an umbrella term for a constellation of conditions associated with the development of cardiovascular disease. They include abdominal obesity; increased triglycerides (stored fat) and low HDL cholesterol; elevated blood pressure; and insulin resistance, which refers to the body's inability to use insulin to properly process sugar.

TM is a simple meditation technique practiced for approximately fifteen to twenty minutes, twice a day, while sitting comfortably with the eyes closed and mentally repeating a mantra. A mantra, chosen by a TM teacher, is a thought sound that has a known vibratory effect but does not have a designated meaning.

Proponents describe it as a simple, natural, easy-to-learn mental technique and believe that regular practice of TM leads to significant cumulative benefits. This occurs on all levels of life, including mind, body, behavior, and environment. More than five million people around the world have learned the technique since it was founded by Maharishi Mahesh Yogi in 1957. It is not considered a religious belief, nor does it conflict with existing religious philosophy.

Lead study author Maura Paul-Labrador, MPH, of Cedars-Sinai Medical Center, Los Angeles, notes that earlier studies found that people who practice TM have lowered their blood pressure, and the study authors wanted to investigate whether the ancient Vedic practice might affect other components of metabolic syndrome.

In the study, fifty-two patients with coronary heart disease were instructed in TM, while fifty-one patients, serving as the control group, received health education. Before the trial and at the end, blood samples were taken from participants after an overnight fast. All participants underwent a medical history review and tests looking at blood vessel function and heart rate variability.

At the end of the sixteen-week study, patients in the meditation group had improved blood pressure and fasting blood-glucose and insulin levels. They also exhibited improved function and stability of the auto-nomic nervous system. The study authors wrote, "These physiological effects were accomplished without changes in body weight, medication, or psychosocial variables and despite a marginally statistically significant increase in physical activity in the health education group." In other words, the study shows these results would have been attained without any changes in body weight, medication, or exercise.

As I mentioned, I engage in the practice of yoga and meditation, and there is scientific proof many of these techniques work. For example, in a controlled trial, the art of tai chi, meditation, walking, exercise, and quiet reading all resulted in similar biochemical and psychological improvements in the response to a stressful experience. In another study reported in the *Journal of Psychosomatic Research* in 2001, researchers found that fifteen minutes of meditation twice a day reduced measures of stress in adolescents.

When you combine a coping technique that you enjoy with a sound diet and exercise, you will be well on your way to a fulfilling life, reducing the potentially harmful effects from stress that too often stifle and immobilize us and keep us from reaching our full potential.

My Prescription for Reducing Stress

If you have problems with stress—and if you do not you are in the minority—I strongly recommend that you explore coping methods that focus on the role of thoughts and emotions and their effect on physical health. There are many options to choose from, including biofeedback, relaxation training, tai chi, yoga, and meditation.

When faced with stress, one organ that responds is our brain, a complex organ unusually susceptible to oxidative damage that can be overcome through nutrition and exercise, as you will see in the next chapter.

PART III
The Benefits of Wellness

One obvious payoff that I have emphasized so far is that following my wellness guidelines can help you minimize the risk of contracting debilitating or chronic diseases. While this has been the focus of the book so far, there are other important benefits you can expect. These include

▶ Enhanced brain and cognitive health

▶ Reduction in the rate of the aging process

▶ Improved appearance

All three of these health areas are directly related to aging. I will focus on these wellness benefits in this section of the book.

9

A Healthy Brain

In 2006, when researchers for the MetLife Foundation asked people over the age of fifty-five what they feared most about aging, many were surprised that financial issues, loss of normal activities, and cancer were not foremost in people's minds. It was the fear of Alzheimer's disease that topped the list. This dreaded form of dementia which, among other things, robs people of their memory, outdistanced several other health concerns that survey respondents cited, including diabetes, heart disease, and stroke.

Unfortunately, the survey also found that while more than a third of U.S. adults knew a family member or friend with Alzheimer's, nearly three-quarters of them knew little or nothing about the disease or what causes it.

According to the Alzheimer's Association, 4.5 million Americans have Alzheimer's disease, a number expected to reach 16 million by 2050. "The greatest risk factor in Alzheimer's is age," said Sibyl Jacobson, president and CEO of MetLife Foundation, in a press release when the study was unveiled. "And, as Americans live longer, the threat of Alzheimer's will continue to increase."

The Most Common Neurological Diseases

What used to be known as "senility" is called "dementia" today. Dementia is an umbrella term used to describe the degradation of intellectual abilities, including memory, serious enough to interfere and ultimately curtail normal activities. People with dementia may not be able to dress themselves or eat. They may get frustrated trying to solve problems they formerly were able to tackle with ease. Their personalities may change, and they may become more emotional. They may have problems formulating their thoughts and speaking. They may also become easily agitated or have visions.

Alzheimer's disease is the most common form of dementia. Alzheimer's destroys brain cells, causing problems with memory, thinking, and behavior severe enough to affect work, lifelong hobbies, or social life. Alzheimer's gets worse over time, and it is fatal. Today it is the sixth-leading cause of death in the United States, and there is no cure.

Lapses of memory are normal, especially as we grow older. People with Alzheimer's experience drastic declines in their ability to communicate, learn, think, and reason. These degraded abilities are severe enough to affect a person's ability to work and take part in social activities and family life.

Our Brains, Inside and Out

The human brain is the most complicated human organ. Our brain contains about 10 billion neurons, and over 100 neurotransmitters have been identified, with many more expected to be discovered. Still, despite giant strides in research techniques and technology over the past few decades, what we know about the brain lags behind what we know of other parts of the body.

We all know that misplacing things and forgetfulness becomes more common as we get older. It is perfectly normal that our cognitive abilities, including memory and learning abilities, decline with age. This decline is due to brain shrinkage, a reduction in the number of synapses, and the depletion of neurotransmitters (including dopamine and serotonin) and neurons. The factors researchers suspect contribute to this decline—other than normal aging and genetics—include hormonal changes, untreated hypertension, poor nutrition, alcohol abuse, sedentary lifestyle, and stress. Also, adult onset diabetes, obesity, and other diseases featuring inflammation increase the possibility of developing a form of dementia.

As should be apparent from this list, many of these factors are under our control. The good news, according to an October 2008 report entitled

Environmental Threats to Healthy Aging by the Greater Boston Physicians for
Social Responsibility and Science and Environmental Health, brain decline
can be slowed down by altering our behavior. Improving our diets, daily
exercise, and stress reduction are all proven steps to keep our brains sharp.
And here is some more good news: researchers have discovered that by studying people's brains as they read and perform other tasks, we can create new
neurons, even after reaching adulthood.

MOOD AND ACTIVITIES MAY STAVE OFF DEMENTIA

While it is widely known that genetics, lifestyle, and environmental factors
contribute to dementia, a study finds that two aspects of lifestyle—personal
mood and staying active—play a bigger role than previously thought.

In the study, which appeared in the January 20, 2009, issue of the journal
Neurology, researchers studied more than 500 elderly people for six years.
At the beginning of the study, the average age of the subjects was 83 years.

Participants completed a questionnaire about their personality traits and
lifestyle, including how easily they became distressed, how extroverted they
were, their number of leisurely activities, and the extent of their social networks.

The researchers discovered that among people who were socially isolated,
those who were calm and relaxed were 50 percent less likely to develop
dementia compared with individuals who were distressed. They also found
that among outgoing extroverts, the dementia risk was 50 percent lower for
people who were calm compared with those who were prone to distress. By
the end of the six years, 144 of the subjects developed dementia.

Researcher Hui-Xin Wang of the Karolinska Institute in Stockholm, Sweden,
said that earlier studies found that chronic distress can affect parts of the brain
such as the hippocampus, possibly leading to dementia, but these new findings
suggest that having a calm and outgoing personality in combination with a
socially active lifestyle may decrease the risk of developing dementia even more.

The good news, the researchers concluded, is that people can control their
levels of activity and mood.

Experience Counts

We do learn to compensate as we get older. Brain scans show that while young people perform certain tasks using only one side, or hemisphere, the brains in older individuals compensate by using both hemispheres. Also, experience counts. Accumulated knowledge—learned skills and experience—can often compensate for a loss of brain mass. This means, explains Denise C. Park, PhD, who in August 2008 was named the T. Boone Pickens Distinguished Chair in Clinical Brain Science at the University of Texas in Dallas, that even when our brain is less efficient at performing complex tasks, our learned experiences, knowledge, and judgment provide a counterbalance.

Food and Our Brains

Eating well is one key to a healthy brain. A professor of neurosurgery and physiological science at the University of California, Los Angeles, believes that a person's diet can improve his or her cognitive abilities and shield the brain from deterioration, including aging. Fernando Gómez-Pinilla, a self-professed fish lover, has analyzed more than 160 studies of food's effect on the brain. Results of his research appeared in *Nature Reviews Neuroscience* and were reported in the July 17, 2008, issue of *The Economist* magazine.

Researchers at Rush University Medical Center in Chicago concur. They have found that people who eat fish at least once a week were 60 percent less likely to develop Alzheimer's disease than were those who did not eat fish.

In addition to seafood, Gómez-Pinilla suggests that people eat more antioxidant-rich foods for their brain's sake because it is susceptible to oxidative damage, it consumes a lot of energy, and the reactions that release this energy generate oxidizing chemicals. Also, brain tissue contains a great deal of oxidizable material, particularly in the fatty membranes surrounding nerve cells.

Although the mechanism by which antioxidants work in the brain is not well understood, Dr. Gómez-Pinilla says it is likely that they protect the synaptic membranes. Synapses are the junctions between nerve cells, and their action is central to learning and memory. But they are also, he says, the most fragile parts of the brain. And many of the nutrients associated with brain function are known to affect transmission at these junctions.

SCIENTIFIC PROOF THAT EXERCISE CAN AID MEMORY

If you want your mind to stay sharp, you need to exercise. Studies published in 2008 found that mild age-related memory loss and dementia—including Alzheimer's—can be delayed by regular physical activity.

In one study, University of North Carolina (UNC) brain researchers discovered that older adult humans who regularly exercised had increased blood flow in their brains. In the study, researchers compared long-time exercisers with sedentary adults using 3-D MRI brain-scanning techniques. The researchers found that active adults had more small blood vessels and improved cerebral blood flow.

During the same period as the UNC study, researchers at Columbia University Medical Center found that levels of blood sugar (glucose) have a direct effect on blood flow in the brain. In this study, researchers tested 240 elderly volunteers using functional magnetic resonance imaging (fMRI). The scientists found a correlation between elevated blood glucose levels and decreased cerebral blood flow in the dentate gyrus, an area in the brain's hippocampus that has a direct effect on our memories. These results correspond with the UNC study.

It is becoming widely accepted that exercise-induced neurotrophins such as brain-derived neurotropic factor (BDNF), vascular endothelial growth factor (VEGF), and the neurotransmitter dopamine are needed to grow new and existing neurons and their synapse connections. These and a host of other recent studies show that exercise-induced blood flow facilitates this process.

One antioxidant Gómez-Pinilla singles out—vitamin E, which is found in vegetable oils, nuts, and green leafy vegetables—has been linked in animal studies with the retention of memory into old age and also with longer life.

Gómez-Pinilla also singles out an omega-3 fatty acid called docosahexaenoic acid (DHA), which helps membranes at synaptic regions transport signals. It also improves a synapse's capacity to change, which can aid memory.

According to the studies reviewed by Dr. Gómez-Pinilla, the benefits of omega-3s include improved learning and memory, and resistance to depression and bipolar disorder, schizophrenia, dementia, attention-deficit disorder, and dyslexia. Omega-3s are found in oily fish, such as salmon, as well as in walnuts, flax seeds, and some fruits.

Gómez-Pinilla offers a word of caution—do not overdo it. Overeating puts oxidative stress on the brain and risks reversing the benefits.

Folic Acid and Dementia

In another study appearing in the British medical journal *The Lancet,* researchers found that folic acid supplements can help people between the ages of 50 and 70 ward off cognitive decline. Also, in a study lasting three years, researcher Jane Durga of Wageningen University in the Netherlands said the study found that people taking folic acid improved their performance when tested on their information-processing speed, ability to memorize, and verbal skills.

The Alzheimer's Association points out that studies show that elevated blood levels of the protein building block homocysteine may increase a person's risk of developing Alzheimer's disease. Other studies have shown that people with Alzheimer's disease often have relatively significant deficiencies in folic acid and vitamin B12 and have subsequently high blood levels of homocysteine. Because homocysteine levels are regulated in part by the body's use of vitamin B12 and folic acid, these findings suggest a possibility that vitamin B12 and folic acid supplements may help lower the risk of developing Alzheimer's disease. Ongoing studies are investigating this possible link.

Exercise and Cognitive Health

In one of the first studies to explore the relationship between cardio-respiratory fitness and the affect on Alzheimer's disease, researchers found that subjects with mild Alzheimer's disease who increased their fitness activities developed more brain mass than mild Alzheimer's patients who exercised less. Results of the study appeared in *Neurology,* the medical journal of the American Academy of Neurology.

For the study, the researchers recruited 121 people age sixty and older who underwent fitness tests using a treadmill and brain scans to measure the total volume of their brains and the amount of white matter and gray matter, two of the three main solid components of the central nervous system. Fifty-seven of the subjects were in the early stages of Alzheimer's disease, while the rest of the members of the study group had no Alzheimer's symptoms.

Study author Jeffrey M. Burns, MD, of the University of Kansas School of Medicine in Kansas City, said the study found that the subjects who were less physically fit with early Alzheimer's disease had four times more brain shrinkage when compared to normal older adults than did those who were more physically fit. Burns said this suggests that higher fitness levels from regular exercise results in less brain shrinkage, even when the Alzheimer's disease process has started, meaning a slower progression of the disease.

"People with early Alzheimer's disease may be able to preserve their brain function for a longer period of time by exercising regularly and potentially reducing the amount of brain volume lost," Burns concluded. "Evidence shows decreasing brain volume is tied to poorer cognitive performance, so preserving more brain volume may translate into better cognitive performance."

Burns said the results remained consistent even when age, gender, severity of dementia, physical activity, and frailty were factored in. However, he cautions that the study only measured fitness levels at one point in time, and further studies are needed to confirm the results.

Exercise and Memory for All Ages

A recent study published in *Behavioral Neuroscience* focused on the question of how to improve memory function as we age. In the study, Yale neuroscientists divided female mice into three age groups: young, middle-aged, and old adults (about three, fifteen, or twenty-one months old, respectively).

The mice were randomly divided into four types of situations:

- ▶ A bare control cage.

- ▶ An exercise group that was provided with running wheels.

- ▶ A group with toys for cognitive stimulation.

- ▶ Cages with both toys and running wheels.

The animals were tested before and during the four-week study, using a common testing tool called the spatial water maze. This test of learning and memory focuses on the hippocampus, which is one of the first areas of the brain to be affected by aging and dementia. All the mice had loss of spatial memory (memory responsible for recording information about one's environment) as they aged.

The researchers found that exercise alone statistically improved the memory of the young mice. Both the exercise and complex environment (toys and running wheels) groups, but not the cognitive stimulation one, improved the memory of the middle-aged mice.

The older mice responded to all enrichment types (alone or in combination) in improving their memory. The complex enrichment resulted in the most benefit for memory.

Other studies have shown that complex enrichment increases brain neuron size, the number of neurons, and the size of the synaptic contact area. In addition, exercise increases the vascular flow to the brain, improving memory.

This suggests that as we get older and unable to exercise as well, cognitive stimulation can help maintain some of the memory. It was even pointed out in the study that complex enrichment at any age could significantly improve memory function.

These studies illustrate that exercise is a key factor in delaying memory loss. There have been numerous studies confirming that thirty to forty minutes of exercise a day slows the aging process of the brain.

My Prescription for a Healthy Brain

Our brains, like all other organs, need care and maintenance. There are a number of things you can do to help keep your brain functioning at its optimal level and to ward off dementia. Here are a few suggestions.

Physical exercise—In addition to strong muscles and endurance, regular exercise keeps nutrition and oxygen flowing to the brain and encourages the growth of new brain cells. By contrast, poor blood circulation is a leading cause of dementia. Also, keeping your weight, blood pressure, cholesterol, and blood sugar levels within recommended ranges all improve brain health.

**CONTRASTING ALZHEIMER'S AND
NORMAL AGE-RELATED MEMORY CHANGES**

Someone with Alzheimer's disease symptoms	Someone with normal age-related memory changes
Forgets entire experiences	Forgets part of an experience
Rarely remembers later	Often remembers later
Is gradually unable to follow written/spoken directions	Is usually able to follow written/spoken directions
Is gradually unable to use notes as reminders	Is usually able to use notes as reminders
Is gradually unable to care for self	Is usually able to care for self

SOURCE: The Alzheimer's Association

Mental exercise—Keeping your brain engaged and challenged maintains and builds reserves of brain cells and new connections. Reading, writing, crossword puzzles, and other mentally challenging activities are all brain-stimulating activities. Even seemingly small things like driving to work via a different route or combing your hair or brushing your teeth with your nondominant hand can help keep your brain sharp.

Diet—Eat a low-fat, low-cholesterol diet that features lean meat, vegetables, and fruits rich in antioxidants, including vitamins E, C, and B-12; folate; and omega-3 fatty acids. A sound diet, along with exercise, is critical for keeping your mind nimble and sharp.

Use caution—To prevent head injuries, use your car's seat belts and wear a helmet when cycling or snow skiing/boarding.

Reduce your stress—Stress and worry are enemies of our mental well-being. While it has never been conclusively proven that reduced levels of stress hormones help maintain healthy brain function, studies show that stress harms the brains of laboratory animals. Consider yoga or meditation, and do whatever helps you to maintain a sense of control over your life.

IF YOU THINK YOU MAY BE DEVELOPING ALZHEIMER'S

The Alzheimer's Association has developed a ten-item checklist to help people recognize the difference between normal age-related memory changes and warning signs of Alzheimer's disease:

1. Memory loss
2. Difficulty performing familiar tasks
3. Problems with language
4. Disorientation to time and place
5. Poor or decreased judgment
6. Problems with abstract thinking
7. Misplacing things
8. Changes in mood or behavior
9. Changes in personality
10. Loss of initiative

Education—It is never too late to enroll in adult education classes and learn new skills.

Stay connected to other people—Leisure activities that combine physical, mental, and social elements may be most likely to prevent dementia. Find activities you enjoy that include other people.

Avoid unhealthy habits—Do not smoke or drink alcohol excessively.

Be creative—It is never too late to develop new hobbies. If you ever had a desire to paint, write, or explore other creative outlets, why not start now?

Attitude is key—It is also very important to stay positive. A study conducted at Rush University Medical Center in Chicago found that people who are often stressed or depressed are 40 percent more likely to develop memory problems than are people with positive attitudes. Based on my experience, patients who undergo surgery with a positive attitude have a better chance of handling the stress, and recovery occurs more quickly and with fewer complications.

If you follow my recommendations in Part II of this guidebook, you can dramatically decrease your chances of developing dementia or you can slow the progression of the disease if it occurs.

Besides keeping our brain sharp and humming along, there is no reason for the rest of our bodies to deteriorate unnecessarily as we grow older. After all, aging is not a disease.

10

Aging on Your Own Terms

Before I meet with a patient scheduled for surgery, I review his or her chart and medical records. I also check the patient's age and weight because they are key determinants for anesthesia. Often, I am surprised when I see a patient who looks literally decades older than his or her birthday indicates.

To some, chronic diseases and body deterioration are thought of as inevitable consequences of aging. To a certain extent, this is true because none of us will live forever. However, when we proactively manage the factors of aging that are under our control, we increase the possibility that we can extend the amount of time that we enjoy good health.

Chronological age is merely a benchmark, and aging does not have to mean spiraling physical decline and chronic illness. We all know thirty-year-olds who look fifty and sixty-year-olds who look forty. And we certainly know adults who act like teenagers. Aging is one of science's biggest mysteries.

Unlocking the Secrets of Aging

Researchers around the world are investigating the biological causes of aging. Every day, they are discovering important new clues about longevity and how to prevent or delay diseases that become more common as we age. This information may not only increase longevity, but also what is known as active life expectancy—the amount of time spent free of disability. Active life expectancy is also popularly referred to as healthspan. The good news, according to the National Institute on Aging (NIA), is that in the last twenty years, the rate of disability among older people has declined dramatically.

While much research in this area remains a mystery, one thing scientists agree on is that aging depends on many processes all contributing to our health and life-span. Our individual genetic makeup, environment, culture, behavior, and lifestyle all contribute to wide variations in the aging of biological processes and systems within the body.

Here are some of the key influences of the aging process.

Aging at the Cellular Level

Most cells have a limited life-span; after a certain number of cell divisions, this ability first slows and then their capacity to divide and synthesize DNA is blocked. This built-in limit on cell division is believed to be a critical factor of the aging process. This complex process, known as senescence, involves a myriad of chemical and physical reactions. Without senescence, organisms could attain some degree of immortality.

Several genes have been identified that regulate senescence; some of them trigger cell proliferation, while others counteract cell division. Research into what causes cells to lose the ability to reproduce and ultimately die could unlock the underlying roots of disease.

Genes and Aging

Recent studies of centenarians have found that longevity runs in families, and genetic influence on life-span is no longer questioned. However, we are still a ways from understanding exactly how and why we age.

Researchers are investigating genetic influences on biological factors associated with extended longevity in animal subjects. Within the last ten years, numerous genes have been discovered that affect normal aging processes, age-related diseases, and other factors associated with the dramatic extension of life-span in worms, fruit flies, and laboratory animals. For example, researchers have bred fruit flies that live nearly twice as long as normal by altering their genes.

Because the human genome is much more complex, advances in genetic research have moved much more slowly. Presently, the National Institute on Aging is confident that exciting discoveries are coming and is underwriting research to discover additional age and longevity-related genes, and is investigating how they relate to body deterioration. For now, altering our genes to extend life is beyond our control.

In addition to genetic influences on aging, there are environmental factors such as toxins, radiation, and free radicals that are produced as cells turn food and oxygen into energy. Progress is being made in understanding and counteracting these environmental effects.

As I have stressed throughout this book, lifestyle choices—eating habits, physical activity, the handling of stress, and other behavioral and social factors such as tobacco use and excessive alcohol consumption—have a profound effect on how we age. All these factors are under our control and have a significant effect on our healthspan.

Calorie Restriction May Lengthen Life

Laboratory research dating back to the 1930s confirms that laboratory animals, when placed on a severely calorie-restricted diet, lived 50 percent longer than the oldest members of their community. There is a growing body of evidence that limiting the amount of food consumed slows the aging process and, as a result, can extend life. Preliminary findings of the Comprehensive Assessment of Long-Term Effects of Reducing Intake of Energy (CALERIE) study at Tufts University in Boston show that adults cutting their calorie consumption by 25 percent lowered their fasting insulin levels and core body temperature, two factors that were shown to increase life span in earlier animal studies. Similar studies are being conducted by the National Institute on Aging, Harvard University, and Washington University.

One obvious advantage of cutting calories is decreasing your chances of weight gain. However, drastically reducing your caloric intake on your own does have pitfalls. For example, a 2006 article in *Archives of Internal Medicine* reports that without exercise, restricting calories may lead to bone density loss.

A one-year study of forty-six participants at Washington University School of Medicine, St. Louis, conducted by Dennis T. Villareal, MD, found that while individuals in a calorie-restricted group did in fact lose weight, they also lost an average of 2.2 percent of their bone density in the lower spine, 2.2 percent at the hip, and 2.1 percent at the top of the femur, all high-risk areas for fracture.

It is important that when cutting calories, you do not do it at the expense of sound nutrition. When planning your meals, you should always include fruits, vegetables, and lean meat to garner the nutrition your body needs. It is a good idea to seek guidance from a dietician or health practitioner with training or experience in nutrition.

Aging and Free Radicals

As I discussed in an earlier chapter, oxygen free radicals are known to attack proteins, cell membranes, and DNA, which can in turn cause aging. Because the body cannot manufacture antioxidants, these very important molecules need to come from our diet and the appropriate nutritional supplements. We now know that to minimize free-radical damage—which can cause premature aging—we need to include an adequate daily supply of antioxidants in our diet. There are two categories of antioxidants: water soluble, such as vitamin C, and fat soluble, such as vitamins A and E.

In humans, vitamin C is the most abundant water-soluble antioxidant. It acts primarily in cellular fluid and has a synergistic relationship with vitamin E. Vitamin C exists in its natural form in a variety of fruits and vegetables, including citrus fruits, berries, broccoli, and peppers.

Vitamin A and beta-carotene (inactive precursor form of vitamin A) are essential for vision and maintaining the health of the mucous membranes that line our various body cavities. Vitamin A is best when consumed from the diet rather than from supplements, to achieve maximum health benefits.

REDUCING ACHES AS YOU AGE

The pain most people associate with getting older is not inevitable. While it is impossible to eliminate skeletal pain totally, you can take some preemptive measures and live the rest of your life relatively pain free.

When older adults complain about pain, their discomfort generally starts with weight-bearing joints, particularly the knees. The knees are placed under tremendous stress with every step, but you can reduce that load one pound at a time. Researchers reporting in the journal *Arthritis & Rheumatism* found that for every pound of weight lost there is a four-pound reduction in the load placed on the knee joint with each step. The accumulated reduction in knee load for a one-pound loss in weight would be more than 4,800 pounds per mile walked. Lose ten pounds, and your knees would be subjected to 48,000 less pounds of pressure per mile. The lesson is simple: less pressure, less knee pain, and the greater amount of exercise a person can perform.

Consider these goals:

- Lose one pound a week by taking in 250 fewer calories and expending an extra 250 calories per day.
- Include strength, aerobic, and stretching activities in your exercise program.
- Ask your doctor if it is okay to try glucosamine/chondroitin supplements to reduce joint pain.

Vitamin A is found in a variety of dark green and deep orange-colored fruits and vegetables such as carrots, sweet potatoes, pumpkin, spinach, butternut squash, turnip greens, mustard greens, and varieties of lettuce, especially romaine.

Vitamin E is the most abundant fat-soluble antioxidant in the body and is one of the most efficient antioxidants available. It is also a primary defender against fat oxidation.

Hormonal Changes

Hormones—the body's chemical messengers, secreted by our glands, that stimulate various functions within the body—are involved in metabolism, immune function, growth, and reproduction. This is an important area of aging research because it has long been known that some hormones decline as we age. For example, growth hormone levels decline, as do levels of the sex hormones; testosterone in males, and estrogen in females. One obvious example of this is the decline of ovarian hormones that accompanies menopause.

Researchers are finding that when reduced levels of certain hormones are replenished by diet and supplementation, some signs of aging diminish. Estrogen replacement therapy after menopause not only alleviates unpleasant menopausal symptoms, but also slows down the accelerated loss of bone seen in osteoporosis. In addition, estrogen replacement therapy may help prevent cardiovascular disease, and there is evidence that it may have a positive effect on brain function.

However, estrogen supplementation is not without controversy. In 2002, researchers with the Women's Health Initiative (WHI) study reported that using estrogen plus progestin may increase the risk of developing heart disease, stroke, blood clots, and breast cancer for some postmenopausal women while also decreasing their risk of hip fractures and colorectal cancer. Two years later, WHI found similar results in postmenopausal women who used estrogen alone.

In 2007, a closer analysis of WHI results found that women aged fifty to fifty-nine at the start of the trial, who used estrogen alone, had significantly less plaque in their coronary arteries (a risk factor for heart attacks) than did women not using estrogen.

Unfortunately, the estrogen replacement controversy has been ongoing for several years and likely will not be settled in the near future.

Overall, research has not shown that any hormone supplements prevent age-related frailty or add years to life. While some supplements benefit people with hormone deficiencies due to a disease or disorder, they also can cause harmful side effects. The body maintains a delicate balance between the amount of each hormone it produces and how much it needs to function properly. It is virtually impossible for hormone supplements to duplicate the body's natural control. This is definitely an area in which people should seek medical advice and supervision.

The ability of the immune system to protect people from infection also declines with age. Several researchers have focused on understanding the complex defense systems the immune system deploys against invading pathogens, coupled with the interactions of hormones and the immune system.

Researchers believe preventing immune system decline could significantly extend the healthspan and quality of life as people age. New discoveries in this area of research will have broad implications for battling infectious diseases, which are a major cause of death for older people.

The Role of Attitude

Obviously, health and aging can be affected by how conscientious a person is in eating well and exercising. But no one can make a person do either. Personality factors also have been shown to have a significant impact on health and aging. For example, people with personalities prone to high anxiety and other negative emotions can suffer from stress, which induces the manufacture of neurotransmitters—messengers of the nervous system—and hormones designed to aid the body in responding to dangerous or stressful situations. When activated at levels above normal on a consistent basis, these hormones can damage cells, tissues, and systems in the body.

Sensory Deterioration

Changes in sensory function—including vision, hearing, taste, smell, and balance—can lead to multiple health and functional problems and may significantly decrease the quality of life for older persons. Relatively simple lifestyle changes can lower the risk of these debilitating factors. For example, not smoking and living in a smoke-free environment can lower the risk of hearing loss, and wearing plastic lenses or hats with brims can reduce cataract risk by lowering eye exposure to ultraviolet light (UVB) from sunlight. Also, wearing earplugs when in an

HEALTHY PAST 100

The Okinawa Centenarian Study, the world's longest-running population-based study of centenarians (now in its twenty-ninth year) reveals a broad range of lifestyle characteristics that contribute to robust health well into later years. The study concentrates on genetics, diet, exercise habits, and psycho-spiritual beliefs and practices.

The researchers report that Okinawans typically are optimistic, adaptable, and easygoing, verifying that attitude is important. They also value spirituality and social engagement. They practice sound eating habits, consuming a diet rich in vegetables, fiber, flavonoids, and good fats, including omega-3s. In addition, they stay lean throughout their lives, eating a low-calorie, low-glycemic load diet and limiting food intake in a cultural practice known as *hara hachi bu,* meaning literally "stomach 80 percent full." They also keep physically active with a variety of daily activities. Compared to North Americans, they have lower rates of dementia, certain cancers such as breast and prostate, osteoporosis, and cardiovascular disease.

Similarly, the New England Centenarian Study at Boston Medical Center also points to certain activities and characteristics. Its Predictors of Reaching 100 list notes that few centenarians are obese and that substantial smoking history is rare. A preliminary study suggests that centenarians are better able to handle stress than the majority of people.

Good genes do help. The New England study found that at least half of centenarians have parents, siblings, or grandparents who had also achieved very old age.

environment with loud noises and opting for headphones rather than earbuds when listening to music can help preserve hearing.

My Prescription for Successful Aging

Aging is not a disease. We need to physically exercise daily, mentally stimulate our minds, and provide our bodies with the proper diet to maintain our memory and maximize the quality of our lives. While my prescription has focused on preventing disease and disability, similar factors can contribute to successful aging—not simply avoidance of disease, but achieving full potential and vitality in later years.

Research into behaviors and health promotion strategies—such as diet, supplements, exercise (including of the brain), and stress reduction—can not only slow premature aging, but can allow you to enjoy life more as you get older. If you eat right and stay active, aging will be nothing to fear.

Nothing shows our age more than our appearance—especially our skin, as you will see in the next chapter.

11

Looking Your Best

A side from the many health benefits you will experience by following the wellness recommendations in this book, there is one benefit that I know everyone will be interested in—looking good. Improvement in appearance, with healthy and youthful-looking hair, skin, and nails, is one of the greatest payoffs from my wellness program. It is the icing on the cake of my recommendations.

Over the years, patients at The Wellness Center have inquired about the effects that nutrition, exercise, and nutritional supplementation will have on their appearance. And why wouldn't they be interested? Having a healthy and youthful appearance is not just a superficial concern. Our outward appearance is a visual and physiologic representation of how healthy we are on the inside. Like other organs in the body, the health of the skin is dependent on optimal care and feeding. Unlike our other organs, we can visualize the skin without any sophisticated scans or monitoring equipment. So, it makes sense that how well we take care of ourselves on the inside will ultimately have an impact on our outward appearance.

Because many health issues and concerns are multifactorial, my approach for achieving optimal health recommends addressing problems from different angles. This certainly holds true for skin health. In fact, I advocate a bidirectional approach, which combines professional skin care products with nutrients and selected nutritional supplements to ensure a healthy, radiant complexion.

Skin Physiology and Function

The skin—which is the largest organ in the body—is not just there for appearance's sake; it has several important functions. The skin protects vital organs, regulates body temperature, acts as a barrier against microorganisms, excretes waste, transforms sunlight into vitamin D, and produces melanin to minimize damage from the sun's ultraviolet rays.

Three layers comprise the skin: the epidermis, dermis, and adipose tissue. The outermost epidermis is the part we see. This epidermal (meaning above the dermis) layer, which is made up primarily of dead cells, protects the skin from the environment. Also, melanin production takes place in the epidermis to protect the skin from ultraviolet light. The middle layer of the skin is the dermis, and the deepest layer is the adipose or fat layer.

If you have ever noticed a baby's skin, it is plump and full. When you gently press it, the skin bounces back immediately. At such a young age, the skin has an abundant supply of three important dermal compounds: collagen, elastin, and hyaluronic acid. Each of these elements is located in the dermis and has the following functions:

- ▶ **Collagen**—responsible for skin firmness

- ▶ **Elastin**—provides the skin's elasticity and resilience

- ▶ **Hyaluronic Acid**—a type of glycosaminoglycan (GAG)—chains of sugars, sulfur, and amino acids that help the skin retain moisture and stay hydrated

Also located in the dermis are hair follicles, sweat glands, oil glands, blood vessels, muscle cells, lymph ducts, and nerve fibers. The nerve endings send messages of touch, heat, pressure, pain, cold, and sexual arousal to the brain.

The bottom layer, adipose tissue—comprised of fat cells—cushions the skin and keeps it from sagging. The fat cells also protect us against extreme temperatures and help shape our body and face. Muscle fibers, nerves, blood vessels, and the roots of oil and sweat glands course through this layer.

Aging Skin and Environmental Damage

Healthy-looking skin is characterized as smooth, with a healthy glow, devoid of blemishes, fine lines, wrinkles, and hyperpigmentation. It is also balanced—neither dry nor oily. Since all of us start off with a healthy, youthful-looking complexion, what changes occur over time that contribute to aging?

After 30, most people's skin begins to show signs of aging. Aging skin is characterized by fine lines and wrinkles. Blemishes may become more pronounced. Usually by age forty, our skin starts to sag, and folds may appear due to fat loss and gravity. This also can cause jowls, droopy eyelids, and horizontal lines across the forehead. Signs of skin aging become even more pronounced as we reach our fifties and sixties.

For postmenopausal women, the outer layer of skin takes longer to renew itself, and the collagen and elastin in the dermal layer continues to break down. A thinning dermis causes wrinkles and furrows, and the skin becomes more transparent.

Aging or senescence is dictated to a large extent by our genetic makeup but also by the normal aging process as I discussed in Chapter 10. As we age, our body's ability to keep up with development, maintenance, and repair is more challenging. In our joints, we are not as efficient at rebuilding and repairing cartilage. In the dermis, we are not as efficient at building new collagen, elastin, and hyaluronic acid.

While multiple theories exist, studies have indicated that the primary cause of aging is related to free-radical production. An editorial appearing in the *New England Journal of Medicine* in 1997 reported that more than 80 percent of facial aging may be caused by exposure to ultraviolet (UV) radiation from the sun; this process is known as photoaging. Free-radical production can cause deterioration of the skin's support structures, decreasing elasticity and resilience and adding to the appearance of aging. Free radicals can also activate the metalloproteinase enzyme, which breaks down collagen.

A steak analogy should help to clarify the last point. An uncooked steak is somewhat difficult to cut into. But once the meat has been placed on a grill and cooked to a medium-well temperature, it is much easier to cut with a knife. The heat helps to release the protein bonds—collagen and elastin—in the meat. It is the same with skin. When these two dermal proteins are cooked in the sun (e.g., tanning), their bonds become unlinked. The decoupling of these protein bonds creates wrinkles. As a result, there is now a multibillion dollar industry to counteract them.

You Are What You Eat

There are a number of well-designed studies on nutrition conducted each year by universities and the National Institutes of Health. These studies, which focus on the role nutrition plays in a wide variety of health issues, including skin health, are not as widely publicized or read as those conducted on pharmaceutical drugs.

Given that your dermatologist may not have mentioned the latest research findings, I have highlighted a few nutrients that hold promise in keeping the skin more youthful. In reviewing the information, you will notice that many of these nutrients function as antioxidants. Antioxidants are the cornerstone of an age management program, and when combined both topically and orally, their effect is more pronounced.

Carotenoids

In a study published in the *American Journal of Clinical Nutrition,* researchers found that the combination of carotenoids plus vitamin E protected against ultraviolet light-induced erythema (redness) in healthy volunteers. In another study published in the *British Journal of Dermatology,* doctors found that foods high in beta-carotene appeared to reduce the risk of psoriasis. Carrots are the best known source for beta-carotene, but this fat-soluble compound is also found in other yellow, orange, and green leafy vegetables, including sweet potatoes, broccoli, cantaloupe, winter squash, tomatoes, and lettuce.

Lutein is a carotenoid that is found in dark green, leafy vegetables, including spinach and kale. Within the skin, lutein appears to be deposited in the epidermis and dermis. An emerging area of research is lutein's role in skin health. Lutein protects the skin by absorbing blue light and quenching free radicals that may be produced in the skin after exposure to the light. A study published in 2007 in the *Journal of Skin Pharmacology and Physiology* demonstrated the benefits of administering lutein to healthy women aged twenty-five to fifty. Those in the treatment group had improved skin hydration, skin lipid content, and skin elasticity. They also had enhanced photoprotective activity whether the lutein was taken orally, applied topically, or administered by both routes.

Vitamins C and E

A growing body of research is reporting that topically applied antioxidants can help protect against sun damage, and a combination of antioxidants and sunscreen provide increased protection. Research appearing in the *Journal of the American Academy of Dermatology* and the *Journal of Investigative Dermatology* reported that, when used in conjunction with sunscreen, vitamins C and E were found to offer photoprotective effects. Specifically, vitamin E showed a boost in UVB protection, and vitamin C offered stronger protection against UVA radiation.

The *Journal of Investigative Dermatology* reported in February 2005 that researchers found a reduction of factors linked to DNA damage within skin cells, leading them to conclude that antioxidant vitamins help protect against DNA damage. Of particular importance are citrus fruits and vegetables rich in vitamin C such as bell peppers, broccoli, cauliflower, and leafy greens.

Pycnogenol®

Pycnogenol is extracted from the bark of the French maritime pine tree. The extract possesses a broad spectrum of biological, pharmacological, and therapeutic activities against free radicals and oxidative stress. In a study published in 2004 in *Free Radical Biology and Medicine,* researchers found that Pycnogenol selectively binds to collagen and elastin and protects these proteins from degradation.

Green Tea Extract

Although green tea has been used in the Orient for centuries, its extract is increasingly recognized in the West for its numerous health-promoting benefits. Green tea contains protective compounds called polyphenols that have antioxidant activity and work as chemopreventive agents. Chemoprevention is the use of chemical agents to prevent the development of cancer. The main green tea polyphenol associated with chemopreventive benefits is epigallocat-echin-3-gallate (EGCG). In experimental studies with human skin, green tea polyphenols demonstrated anti-inflammatory and anticarcinogenic properties.

Alpha-Lipoic Acid

This powerful antioxidant is hundreds of times more potent than either vitamin C or E. Alpha-lipoic acid helps neutralize skin cell damage caused by free radicals, much like vitamins C and E. Alpha-lipoic is a versatile antioxidant in that it works in both fat-soluble and water-soluble environments. In one study conducted at Yale University and published in the *Archives of Gerontology and Geriatrics* in 1999, researchers found that alpha-lipoic acid protected proteins against damage by free radicals.

Essential Fatty Acids

Our bodies require a number of essential nutrients to promote and maintain health. Although some dietary fats are considered harmful, two special types of fat are necessary for good health and youthful skin. These two fats (or fatty acids) must be obtained either through diet or supplementation, hence their name: essential fatty acids EFAs). Both EFAs are polyunsaturated fats with one member, alpha-linolenic acid, belonging to the omega-3 family and the other, linoleic acid, belonging to the omega-6 family.

EFAs perform a number of vital functions in the body but are particularly important at the cellular level because they are a fundamental component of the membranes of all cells. An adequate supply of EFAs in the diet is also essential for healthy-looking skin because skin cells turn over very rapidly.

A study published last year in the *British Journal of Nutrition* demonstrated that skin properties can be modulated by an intervention with dietary lipids. Healthy women volunteers who took flaxseed oil for twelve weeks had significant increased skin hydration, decreased transepidermal water loss, and a significant decrease in skin roughness and scaling compared to the control group.

In another study published in 2007 in the *American Journal of Clinical Nutrition*, researchers found that better skin-aging appearance among middle-aged women was associated with higher intakes of vitamin C and linolenic acid. These women had a lower likelihood of a wrinkled appearance, senile dryness (dryness associated with aging), and skin atrophy (thinning skin).

Hyaluronic Acid

Hyaluronic acid is one of the skin's most important components for hydration and moisture retention. The nature of the hyaluronic acid molecular structure makes it ideal for attracting and holding water. Nearly 50 percent of the body's hyaluronic acid is found in the dermis, in the spaces between cells (extracellular matrix). Hyaluronic acid, along with dermatan sulfate, serves to maintain the water balance in the dermis and adds support for other dermal elements like collagen and elastin. As we age, our ability to produce sufficient levels of hyaluronic acid diminishes and, as a result, the skin becomes drier and more vulnerable to damage.

A study published in the *Journal of Investigative Dermatology* examined changes in the deposition of hyaluronan (hyaluronic acid) in human skin with advancing age. No significant differences in hyaluronan concentrations were found in human skin of different ages, but researchers did find that with aging, hyaluronan levels increased in the lower layers of the dermis, while the upper layers of the dermis showed a decline. This observation may explain some of the changes in human skin that occur with aging.

My Prescription for Healthy/Youthful Skin

I recommend that you adopt the following habits every day to maintain healthy, vibrant, and younger-looking skin.

1. **Eat more nutrient-dense whole foods, especially organic vegetables and fruits, every day.** The less processed, the more likely your foods will contain the nutrients and fiber that are vital for the healthy functioning of your body and skin.

2. **Avoid packaged and processed foods.** These foods often contain large amounts of sodium and are made with partially hydrogenated fats/oils. Increasingly, research is demonstrating the negative health effects of dietary sodium and partially hydrogenated fat.

3. **Replace simple carbs with slow carbs.** Refined sugars elevate blood insulin levels, which can have negative long-term health consequences. Replace simple carbs like bagels, pasta, bread, and desserts with ample fruit and vegetable consumption. Learn to shop the perimeter of the food store, where healthier foods are located.

4. **Hydrate your body.** It is important to drink plenty of high-quality water each day. As an organ of elimination, the skin requires ample water to maintain proper function and get rid of toxins.

5. **Exercise regularly—aerobic, resistance, and stretching.** Make sure that you get an adequate balance of aerobic, resistance, or weight training and stretching exercises. Yoga is excellent for both strength and flexibility.

6. **Protect against sun exposure.** One of the symptoms of dermal environmental damage is dryness. In addition to its many other harmful effects, the sun can dry out the skin. Avoid direct sun exposure, and use a moisturizing sunscreen product with adequate SPF for your exposure.

7. **Be aware of facial expressions.** Repetitive facial expressions can cause deep frown lines that contribute to an aged appearance.

8. **If you smoke—stop now.** Aside from all of the health problems smoking creates, this habit looks unattractive, creates wrinkles (especially around the mouth), and causes the skin to look sallow; it also can give the fingernails a yellow tint.

9. **Limit alcohol and caffeine intake.** Both alcohol and caffeine dehydrate the body, contributing to dry skin. Alcohol also interferes with nutrient metabolism and is a factor in capillary fragility and breakage.

10. **Get enough sleep.** Inadequate sleep can lead to skin that looks ashen and contributes to puffiness around the eyes. Be aware of your body position during sleep—optimal is lying supine (on your back).

Conclusion

Every day, we make personal choices and decisions—dozens, if not hundreds of them. Most we do not even think about—which shoe to put on first, whether to turn left or right when driving home from work. Some decisions require a bit more thought—what to wear, which program to watch on TV, or what bills to pay.

Unfortunately, many of the important choices we make—particularly the ones that affect our health—are made haphazardly. For example: what we choose to eat for breakfast or lunch, whether to exercise or not, whether to engage in stressful or risky activities, or whether to take on more than we can handle. All of these daily choices can have unintended but lasting consequences.

Also, too many people ignore their health in order to get ahead. Their jobs, careers, or family-related activities take precedence over everything else. Some seem to subscribe to the philosophy, "It won't happen to me." They somehow believe that they will not be the one who gets cancer or heart disease or other diseases. It is as though they believe they have Teflon bodies that will prevent illness from sticking to them. I have had many, many conversations with patients over the years, trying to understand why they make these poor choices . . . why they eat the way they do . . . why they do not exercise . . . why they just do not seem to value their health.

As part of my wellness evaluation, I ask all patients to create a values list—a list of the things that are important to them. I have them compose a list of the top ten or twelve things they value. Items on the list might include family, security, love, certainty, freedom, health, recognition, or faith. Then I ask them to prioritize the list. They are instructed to list the most important values first and then move down the list in order of priority. This is not an easy exercise for most people. What I often find when I review the values list with patients is that health is not on the list or is very low in priority.

One of the most important pieces of advice I give to patients seeking wellness is to make health a top priority on their values list. Too often, health is ignored until illness rears its ugly head. When our health suffers, all of the other things that are important to us take a back seat. Without our health, it can be difficult or impossible to work, to have fun, to care for our families, and sometimes even to enjoy life.

Personal Responsibility

What is the best way to get started on the road to wellness? A key element is the need for each of us to accept responsibility for our health and well-being. The act of being responsible is a dynamic process. For us to act responsibly, our active participation is required. Too often, people rely on our health care system to provide for their care—and usually it is after problems have occurred.

I think it is a fair assumption that you probably read this book because you are proactive or want to be. After reading the book, my hope is that you will not feel overwhelmed or sense that it might be too difficult or complicated to initiate a wellness-oriented lifestyle. While change is challenging, and it is natural to be somewhat resistant, it is important to remember that we all have the capacity to change.

Over the years, I have seen countless patients at The Wellness Center who have made the decision and commitment to change and lead a healthier lifestyle. I have seen patients who, despite major health challenges, have made significant modifications in their diet and lifestyle. Fortunately, when it comes to health, change does not have to happen all at once. Small, incremental adjustments—made on a day-to-day basis—can have significant and lasting health effects.

Scientific research continues to demonstrate that small changes in diet and daily physical activity can significantly increase a person's life span. One of the leading experts in the field of health and disease, Professor Kay-Tee Khaw, is studying the links between lifestyle and the development of chronic diseases such as cancer. She is currently one of the principal UK scientists working on the European Prospective Investigation into Cancer and Nutrition (EPIC) study. The EPIC study is a European-wide project investigating the links among diet, lifestyle, and cancer.

Khaw's research looks at the life span of various people to find out why some people live longer, healthier lives. She has found that people can gain extra years of life by making small changes. To date, Khaw's studies have looked at over 22,000 people in Norfolk, England, from age forty-five to seventy-nine. Her work illustrates that no matter where in life a person decides to start making lifestyle changes, he or she can improve the chances of living a longer, healthier life.

The studies have proven that just one extra piece of fruit or serving of vegetables a day can contribute to a longer life. Her research also demonstrates that moderate amounts of activity, like walking up the stairs instead of taking an elevator, can lengthen someone's life. This work demonstrates that these changes not only increase life span but are also related to better quality of life.

Doctor–Patient Communication

When I speak with patients, one issue they commonly voice is their confusion about health information. Granted, media health reports can be conflicting and confusing. One month a low-fat diet is recommended, the next the headlines indicate that a low-fat diet is unhealthy. Because of this lack of clear information, many patients decide to do nothing. This is unfortunate.

Nowadays, a vast amount of solid health information is available, particularly on the internet. While some of this information is hype, excellent information is obtainable on Web sites sponsored by institutions, including the National Institutes of Health. (I've provided a list of trustworthy sites at the end of the bibliography.)

More than anything, it is important that you find a health care provider you trust. And when you do, it is essential to ask questions. It is also just as important that you understand your doctor's answers. Some people are intimidated by physicians; some think the doctor's time is too valuable, and others think they're being impolite if they ask too many questions. I suspect many of us are more inquisitive with our car mechanics and appliance service people than with our health care providers.

The U.S. Health and Human Services' Agency for Healthcare Research and Quality (AHRQ) initiated a program in 2007 to convince people to be more involved in their health care. They compiled a checklist of questions people should ask their doctors. Here is a sample of what AHRQ suggests:

▶ You know important things about your symptoms and your health history. Tell your doctor what you think he or she needs to know.

▶ It is important to tell your doctor personal information—even if it makes you feel embarrassed or uncomfortable.

▶ Bring a health history list with you, and keep it up to date. You might want to make a copy of the form for each member of your family.

▶ Always bring any medicines you are taking or a list of those medicines (include when and how often you take them as well as their strength). Talk about any allergies or reactions you have had to your medicines.

▶ Tell your doctor about any herbal products you use or alternative medicines or treatments you receive.

▶ Bring other medical information, such as X-ray films, test results, and medical records.

▶ Ask questions. Ask the doctor to explain further if you are not sure you understand.

▶ Write down your most important questions before your visit. Make sure they get asked and answered.

▶ Take notes.

In addition to many patients' reluctance to ask questions, I admit, frankly, that doctors are often unwilling to take the time to provide answers. As a physician and someone who has also been a patient, I pass along the following reminders:

You are the reason the doctor is here and not the other way around. It is part of the doctor's job to establish open and effective communication with you. He or she should be receptive to discussion and questions from you. In fact, it is vital that you and your doctor have quality communication so you understand the information and his or her instructions. After all, it is your health and wellness we are talking about. It is important to remember that no one cares more about you than you do, and that is the way it should be.

=Appendix A=

More on the Immune System and Inflammation

O perating behind the scenes, your immune system is made up of a number of interdependent cell types that work together to protect your body. Before a foreign particle can enter the body, it has to get through several barriers, with the skin as the first line of defense. Next, mucous membranes lining the sinus cavities trap many foreign particles, and the villi of the respiratory tract catch even more.

Saliva in the mouth contains enzymes that not only begin the digestive process, but they also destroy pathogens before they are swallowed. Next, stomach acids destroy more foreign particles before they are transported to the intestines. While these mechanisms are very effective in eliminating foreign and potentially damaging material, sometimes pathogens make it into the bloodstream after leaving the digestive tract.

Our bodies have a defense system there also. Coursing through the blood and lymph streams are trillions of T and B cells (roughly one trillion T cells and one trillion B cells). In the lymphoid organs and in the bloodstream, there are approximately 10 billion antigen-presenting cells (APCs), usually macrophages and dendritic cells. By circulating these cells throughout the blood and lymph streams, the body maximizes the chances of finding foreign particles when they enter the body. Any given immune cell may circulate between the blood and lymph systems up to fifty times each day.

When an antigen enters the body, it is usually detected and trapped by APCs. APCs then present the antigen to the lymphocytes in the blood or lymph fluids, and those lymphocytes with receptors specific to that antigen stop it from migrating and initiate a local immune response. Sometimes antigen-presenting cells degrade or even destroy antigens without the help of other immune cells, but if there are too many antigens for the APCs to handle them alone, the APCs secrete a chemical message in the form of interleukin-1 (IL-1). The APCs display fragments of the antigens to the helper T cells that answer the chemical summons.

In especially serious infections, the APCs secrete large amounts of IL-1, often causing fever and drowsiness. The helper T cells that answer the call and encounter fragments of the antigens then transform into lymphoblasts. These new cells secrete new interleukins (especially IL-2 and IL-3), which are essential to a successful immune response. IL-2 stimulates cytotoxic T cells, which may be needed to kill cells with malignant characteristics or cells infected by a virus. IL-3 stimulates the production of blood cells in the bone marrow, ensuring an adequate supply of immune cells and cell products to continue to fight the infection. Helper T cells also secrete interleukins that stimulate B cells to divide and morph into antibody-secreting plasma cells.

In the case of certain tumor cells, messenger cells alert natural killer (NK) cells, which travel to the site and kill abnormally replicating cells. Natural killer cells, if they come in contact with tumor cells, can also kill on their own, without being prompted or stimulated by another immune cell. NK cells are different from other cells of the immune system in that they attack and destroy microbe-infected cells rather than attacking the microbe itself.

The immune response may occur either naturally through infection by a pathogen, or artificially through vaccination. The improved resistance and acquired immune memory gained when the body responds to a foreign antigen is called active immunity. Active immunity—both natural and artificial—lasts longer than passive immunity (immunity transferred from another source, such as antibodies passed to a fetus through the placenta or a gamma-globulin injection) because it uses immune memory gained through experience.

Nearly every organ in the body either plays a role in or is directly affected by the immune response. However, several organs perform particularly important functions.

Bone Marrow: Every immune cell is derived from the bone marrow. Stem cells in the bone marrow differentiate, through a process called hematopoiesis, into mature immune system cells or into cell precursors that travel to other parts of the body to finish maturation. The bone marrow generates natural killer cells, B cells, granulocytes, immature thymocytes, and red blood cells and platelets.

Liver: The liver has more functions than any other organ does, but its role as the primary filter of impurities is especially important to the immune system. As blood passes through, the liver filters out bacteria and other pathogens and produces factors that initiate an immune response.

Lymph Nodes: The lymph system performs three main jobs in the overall immune response: It drains fluid from tissues back into the bloodstream. It detects pathogens and antigens in the fluid by passing it through the lymph nodes, which contain several types of immune cells, and it fights infection.

As blood circulates through the body, a fluid called plasma leaks out and bathes the tissues of the body. This fluid carries food to cells and removes waste products and transports them back to the lymphatic system, which passes it through the spleen and lymph nodes for filtration and detection of pathogens. Then the lymph fluid is passed back into the bloodstream, and the cycle is repeated.

When people who are ill say, "My glands are swollen," they are talking about their lymph nodes, which are inflamed because the white blood cells they contain are fighting infection. The lymphatic system also aids immunity by helping to make white blood cells that produce antibodies. The lymph nodes contain immune blood cells called macrophages, which envelope and kill foreign elements and also produce antibodies that detect and fight infection. These macrophages, along with dendritic cells, present these elements to T and B cells, which then initiate a full immune response.

Spleen: The spleen is one of the body's primary immunologic filters. As blood passes through the spleen, immune cells (B cells, T cells, macrophages, natural killer cells, dendritic cells and red blood cells) capture foreign antigens. An antigen is any foreign substance that evokes an immune response. Cells in the spleen then channel information about the captured antigens to the right cells, which will then produce antibodies and resist the abnormality. The spleen basically serves as a sort of immunological communications hub, where cells come to share information and to initiate an appropriate immune response.

Thymus: The thymus is a small gland located high in the chest behind the breastbone. The main function of the thymus is to produce mature T cells. Immature thymocytes leave the bone marrow and travel to the thymus to mature and to be "educated" about their role in the immune system. During this process, the thymus actually weeds out the T cells that might induce a harmful immune response. Only those T cells that mature properly and learn their job well are released into the bloodstream.

When Things Go Wrong

But what happens when there is miscommunication within this complex process? Any of these scenarios may occur:

▶ If your immune system cells fail to distinguish "self" from "nonself," it can generate an immune response against itself (resulting in an autoimmune disorder, such as lupus).

▶ When the body cannot build appropriate immune responses against invading microorganisms, an immunodeficiency disorder can lead to chronic and even deadly infections.

▶ If what should be a normal immune response to foreign antigens goes overboard and damages normal tissues, you can experience an allergic reaction (including life-threatening anaphylaxis).

Symptoms of Food Allergy

A food allergy is the result of your body's immune system overreacting to food proteins called allergens. For the most part, we develop tolerances to the foods in our diet, and the immune system lets them pass. However, everyone's immune system is different. As part of your body's defense, some immune systems recognize certain foods as dangerous and, in their response to the offending food, cause what we know as allergic reactions.

Allergic reactions to food can last from minutes to hours, and the severity of the reaction varies widely between people. Mild allergic reactions include a runny nose, watery eyes, or sneezing. On the other hand, highly allergic and life-threatening reactions can include asthma attacks, rapid heartbeat, and swelling of the tongue or throat.

The most common symptoms of food allergy involve the skin and digestive system. Skin reactions include hives and eczema. Digestive symptoms may include nausea, vomiting, cramps, and diarrhea.

It is important to know that food allergy symptoms can be caused by a number of different diseases, so it is important to seek medical attention as soon as possible when symptoms appear.

In reaction to a food allergy, the immune system produces increased amounts of immunoglobulin E antibody (IgE), which activates histamine and other chemicals. To maximize their effectiveness, these chemicals may cause blood vessels to widen, smooth muscles to contract, and skin to become red, itchy, and swollen.

More About Inflammation

The Belgian researchers who conducted the study appearing in the September 2005 issue of the *Journal of Occupational and Environmental Medicine* (see Chapter 2) gave a questionnaire to 892 male workers without cardiovascular disease to gauge three suspected components of occupational stress:

▶ Psychological job stress

▶ Job control

▶ Social support (and conflict) at work

The researchers from Ghent University then compared indicators of job stress with levels of known laboratory markers of inflammation and infection.

The researchers found that workers who felt they had little control over their jobs had increased levels of fibrinogen—a blood-clotting factor linked to myocardial infarction and other cardiovascular diseases—regardless of age, occupation, or whether they smoked. They also determined that stress was unrelated to other markers of inflammation, including C-reactive protein (CRP) and serum amyloid A.

Lead researcher Els Clays, MSc, said that they also found little relationship between stress and markers of infection, even though earlier studies linked high stress levels to an increased risk of cardiovascular disease, which could not be attributed to common risk factors such as high blood pressure and cholesterol.

Link Between Obesity and Inflammation

According to a study appearing in *Circulation* in 2006, researchers found that obesity may be associated with chronic inflammation, evidenced by elevated cytokine and chemokine levels and increased macrophage accumulation in fat (adipose) tissue. They also found that T cells, which can play an important role in chronic inflammatory diseases such as atherosclerosis, have not been as well studied in obesity. This study hypothesized that elevated chemokines levels in adipose tissue in obesity are also associated with increased T cell accumulation.

The researchers found that a high fat diet leads fat cells to produce chemokines, which attract inflammatory white blood cells into fat tissue. Specifically, they discovered both macrophages and T cells (which play a critical role in the immune system) accumulate in fat tissue, beginning the process that leads to disease.

There's more. Researchers at Washington University School of Medicine in St. Louis report that fat in the belly may promote inflammation leading to diabetes and heart disease. The researchers found that fat cells inside the abdomen secrete molecules that increase inflammation, establishing a potential link between abdominal fat and inflammation. The researchers concluded that the discovery could be key as scientists learn more about the key role of inflammation in diabetes, heart disease, and other illnesses.

As mentioned earlier in the book, liposuction does not appear to provide the metabolic benefits normally associated with similar amounts of fat loss induced by dieting or exercising. In a study appearing in the March 2007 issue of the journal *Diabetes,* researchers looked instead at visceral fat—the fat that surrounds the organs in the gut. Unlike subcutaneous fat, visceral fat is too close to the intestines and other internal organs to remove surgically. Because they could not remove the fat, the researchers decided to analyze the blood supply that ran through it in twenty-five obese patients to see whether visceral fat was involved in inflammation or if, like subcutaneous fat, it was only a marker of potential problems.

They found that visceral fat in the abdomen was secreting high levels of an important inflammatory molecule called interleukin-6 (IL-6) into blood in the portal vein. The researchers concluded that by contributing to inflammation, visceral fat cells in the abdomen may be doing even more than that.

Several studies suggest that the polyphenols found in fruits and vegetables can relieve inflammation and effectively lower the risk of certain diseases because of their anti-inflammatory capabilities. For example, a 2005 study from a Spanish research team examined the effects of select flavanols extracted from food on the secretion and activity of pro-inflammatory compounds produced by the body's macrophage cells. Normally, the inflammation signals they send are helpful, but if responding to a chronic threat (such as infection or high levels of oxidized fat in the blood vessel walls), the risk of chronic inflammation increases dramatically. The researchers found that flavanols were able to inhibit the production and activity of inflammation-causing cytokines and chemokines.

Inflammation and Heart Disease

Researchers from the University of Nottingham published a study in 2006 investigating the potential of flavonoids in the reduction of inflammation within the cardiovascular system. While other studies have linked this food compound and its potential to reduce the risk of CVD, this study sought to determine a possible mechanism behind the benefit.

Noting that platelets and leukocytes both contribute to inflammatory processes involved in CVD, the researchers gave healthy volunteers a flavanol-rich beverage—in this case cocoa—and tested various markers for inflammation and blood platelet aggregation.

The findings show that the consumption of a flavanol-rich foods also resulted in inhibition of the activation of certain leukocytes and a significant decrease in inflammation markers. The researchers concluded that consumption of these type foods could contribute to a reduced risk of CVD and related conditions.

Another study indicating that flavanols may help suppress the effects of inflammation in cardiovascular disease was published in a 2005 issue of the *American Journal of Clinical Nutrition*. A German research team focused on the effects of catechin and epicatechin—two types of flavanols—on inflammation-causing leukotrienes. The researchers found that the flavanols inhibited the activity of 5-lipoxygenase, the key enzyme in leukotriene synthesis—a key finding in determining the mechanisms behind the flavanols' anti-inflammatory and vascular-protective properties. The findings also confirmed other research showing that flavanols can limit the oxidation of LDL fats, which play a key role in the formation of atherosclerosis and other forms of CVD.

Inflammation and Diarrhea

Scientists have known for some time that inflammation is central to the onset of dangerous gastrointestinal disorders such as dysentery and diarrhea. In fact, infectious diarrhea is the second largest killer of children under the age of five, claiming the lives of more than 2 million children every year. "This neglected disease is devastating, not only because one in 200 children who contract infectious diarrhea will die from it, but for those who survive, it has a lifelong, generation-wide impact," states Victoria Hale, founder of OneWorld Health, a nonprofit organization seeking new treatments to curb the devastation of diarrhea, especially in developing countries.

Social scientists and health experts also know that polyphenols have been used for generations in various cultures as a traditional medicine for diarrhea, dysentery, and related conditions. Science is now catching up to the knowledge of native healers. Research shows that different classes of polyphenols (such as flavanols) are effective at reversing diarrhea, probably through different mechanisms. One study from Canada found that polyphenols in apples protected the epithelial cells that line the digestive tract.

In addition, researchers from Canada and Puerto Rico demonstrated that dysfunction of the epithelial cells in the intestinal tract contributes to chronic inflammation, and thereby various gastrointestinal ailments such as inflammatory bowel syndrome, colitis, and diarrhea. The researchers also determined that an ongoing cycle of chronic inflammation and inflammatory bowel conditions is conducive to the buildup of pathogens—such as diarrhea-causing bacteria—in the intestinal tract.

= Appendix B =

How Free Radicals Form

M aybe a short chemistry–biology refresher course is in order. As you may recall from high school, a structural feature of every cell in our body and which determines chemical behavior is the number of electrons in the outer shell of atoms. Atoms often complete their outer shells by sharing electrons with other atoms. By sharing electrons, the atoms are bound together and stabilize the molecules. Normally, the process works well.

When the bond between atoms weakens, unstable free radicals form. Lacking an electron, free radicals seek and try to capture a nearby electron from another atom to gain stability. When the attacked molecule loses its electron, it also becomes a free radical and seeks an electron to replace it. This oxidative stress can set off a chain reaction within the cell, weakening it and sometimes causing premature death of the cell.

Types of Free Radicals

There are seven different types of free radicals that have been identified.

1. Superoxide anion
2. Hydroxyl radical
3. Hydrogen peroxide
4. Singlet oxygen
5. Polyunsaturated fatty acid radicals
6. Organic fatty acid hydroxyl radicals
7. Oxidized protein

=Appendix C=

Vitamins and Minerals

Vitamins

Vitamins are organic compounds the body needs in very small amounts for normal growth and maintenance of good health. They play important metabolic roles. Our bodies have no mechanism for creating vitamins, so the vitamin molecules must be obtained through the foods and supplements we consume. The human body needs at least thirteen different vitamins to function properly. There are two groups of vitamins: the fat soluble and the water soluble.

Vitamin A: Helps maintain smooth, soft, disease-free skin and helps protect the mucous membranes of the mouth, nose, throat, and lungs, which also helps reduce the risk of infections and protects against air pollutants and other contaminants. It also helps maintain and improve eyesight and counteracts night blindness. It also aids in bone and teeth formation and maintenance; improves skin elasticity, moisture retention and suppleness; and helps reverse the signs of photoaging. A lack of vitamin A can cause skin to become dry and hardened.

Beta-Carotene: Used by the body to produce vitamin A; essential for vision, growth, cell division, reproduction, and immunity.

Vitamin B Complex: B-complex vitamins are a mixture of eight essential B-vitamins that our bodies require daily. Their numbers represent the order in which they were discovered. At one time, it was thought that vitamin B was a single nutrient, but later studies proved that it was actually eight different nutrients. Each of these vitamins performs a unique and separate function in the body. Overall, they help with the metabolism of protein, energy production, brain function, and blood cell formation.

Biotin: Four enzymes critical to metabolism require this water-soluble B vitamin to function properly. Biotin—also known as vitamin H—helps the body break down food and use it for energy and helps metabolize protein, fats, and carbohydrates.

Vitamin B1 (Thiamin): Thiamin is essential for proper carbohydrate metabolism; it also works to improve mood and overcome heartburn. It is used by the body to pump blood in and out of the heart as well as to help prevent diseases that affect the nerves.

Vitamin B2 (Riboflavin): Riboflavin is necessary for red blood cell formation as well as for assisting with fat, protein, and carbohydrate metabolism. It also works to improve skin blemishes and migraines and in preventing the onset of cataracts.

Vitamin B3 (Niacin): Niacin is an effective aid for lowering cholesterol, as well as promoting healthy skin. It can also be used to treat depression, insomnia, and arthritis.

Vitamin B5 (Pantothenic Acid): Pantothenic acid works to promote a healthy central nervous system as well as assist in energy production and fight chronic fatigue, migraines, allergies, and heartburn.

Vitamin B6 (Pyridoxine): Pyridoxine is needed for almost every function in the body, working as a coenzyme for numerous enzymes. It also plays a major role in forming red blood cells, proteins, and neurotransmitters as well as in stabilizing homocysteine levels. Supplemental B6 can be used to relieve PMS and asthma attacks.

Vitamin B9 (Folic Acid): Folate is essential during pregnancy to protect against birth defects; also stabilizes homocysteine levels.

Vitamin B12 (Cyanocobalamin): Cyanocobalamin is essential to prevent pernicious anemia, which is caused by B12 deficiency.

Vitamin C: A powerful antioxidant for fighting free radicals, vitamin C is also necessary for maintaining skin integrity, promoting immune system activity, and protecting red blood cells.

Vitamin D: Known as the sunshine vitamin, vitamin D is actually a hormone that is produced in our bodies by ultraviolet B rays. These light rays trigger the production of vitamin D by our skin cells. The hormone that is produced is called calcitriol, and once it is made, it travels to the intestines to help with the absorption of dietary calcium and fluoride.

Vitamin E: An antioxidant that protects fatty acids and vitamin A from being oxidized. It is also an anti-blood-clotting agent that helps with healthy red blood cell development.

Minerals

Minerals are naturally occurring elements found in the Earth's crust both on land and in the sea. The natural processes of climate and erosion create mineral salts, which are absorbed by plants and are in turn consumed by humans.

Often they work together. For example, magnesium, calcium, and potassium are extremely important in regulating the rhythm of the heart. In fact, deficiencies of any of these important minerals can result in irregular heartbeat, instantly raising the risk of heart disease.

Minerals are categorized as macrominerals or microminerals (trace minerals or elements).

Boron: This trace mineral enhances skeletal mineral absorption and bone density and supports mental alertness.

Calcium: Necessary for strong teeth and bones as well as efficient muscle and nerve function.

Chloride: Chloride works with potassium and sodium, the two electrolytes, to control the flow of fluid in blood vessels and tissues; it regulates acidity in the body and forms part of hydrochloric acid in the stomach.

Chromium: This trace mineral enhances glucose tolerance and modulates fat metabolism as an energy source.

Copper: Copper, along with iron, helps in the formation of red blood cells. It also helps to keep the blood vessels, nerves, the immune system, and bones healthy.

Iodine (Organic): Supports normal metabolism and optimal thyroid function.

Iron: This essential mineral is an important component of proteins involved in oxygen transport and metabolism. Almost two-thirds of the iron in the body is found in hemoglobin, the protein in red blood cells that carries oxygen to body tissues. About 15 percent of iron is stored for future needs and is mobilized when dietary intake is inadequate. The remainder is in body tissues as part of the proteins that help bodily functions.

Magnesium: There is no mineral used by more cells or systems within the human body. Virtually every cell in the human body uses magnesium, and it affects over 300 different enzymes. Magnesium plays an important role in maintaining nerve impulses and nerve function, regulating heart rhythm, and keeping bones strong.

Manganese: This trace mineral is important for energy production, protein and fat metabolism, and numerous growth functions.

Phosphorous: This is the second most abundant element—after calcium—present in our bodies, making up about 1 percent of our total body weight. It is present in every cell, but 85 percent of the phosphorus is found in the bones and teeth. In the bones, phosphorus is present in the phosphate form as the bone salt calcium phosphate. Just like calcium, phosphorous is in constant turnover, even in the bone structure.

Potassium: Potassium is found both inside and outside of our cells. Known as an electrolyte, potassium—along with other minerals such as sodium, chloride, and calcium—is essential for normal cellular function such as conducting nerve impulses; initiating muscle contractions; and helping the body to convert glucose, the primary energy molecule used by the body, into glycogen, the body's stored form of energy.

Selenium: Selenium is an essential trace mineral and is a vital antioxidant enzyme that protects cells. Selenium is also essential for normal functioning of the immune system and the thyroid gland. Selenium also inhibits the oxidation of lipids.

Sodium: The body uses this electrolyte to regulate blood pressure and blood volume. Sodium is also critical for the functioning of muscles and nerves. Too much can contribute to high blood pressure, kidney disease, and other health problems.

Zinc: This mineral is involved in wound healing, the sense of taste and smell, growth, and sexual maturation and is contained in enzymes that regulate metabolism.

Sources: *The American Botanical Council, FDA, USDA, and other NIH sites.*

=Appendix D=

More on Aging

To understand how calorie restriction affects aging, researchers examined 6,500 mouse genes and identified fifty-eight genes that produced or expressed more than twice as much biochemical material as the mice aged. These genes were primarily involved in stress responses and neuron growth, which was of interest because researchers found that caloric restriction produced a heightened stress response after proteins and other large molecules were damaged.

Telomeres—a region of repetitive DNA found at the end of chromosomes—are regarded as the cell's molecular clock. These protective segments shorten each time certain types of cells divide until cell division ceases. In the past few years, major advances have been made in understanding the role telomeres play in cellular life cycles and death.

To date, researchers have learned that the enzyme telomerase compensates for telomere shortening by adding more DNA segments to the ends of chromosomes, enabling cells (including sperm) to divide indefinitely. In one experiment, scientists inserted the gene for telomerase in normal, telomerase-negative cells. As a result, telomeres grew longer, and the cells replicated far beyond known limits for normal cells while retaining the function of younger cells. Scientists say this discovery suggests not only that telomeres are the central timing mechanism for cellular aging but also that the mechanism can be altered.

Scientists believe controlled activation of telomerase may provide an avenue for healthy cell division by resetting or extending the timing mechanisms. Their ultimate goal is to unlock the mechanisms of telomerase activity that lead to cancerous growth and to learn methods to inhibit telomerase growth, developing a new avenue to cure cancer.

Bibliography

Periodicals and Medical Journal Articles

Chapter 1: Behind Today's Health Crisis

DeBoer, S, Thomas, RJ, Brekke, MJ, Brekke, LN, Hoffman, RS, Menzel, PA, Aase, LA, Hayes, SN, Kottke, TE. 2003. Dietary intake of fruits, vegetables, and fat in Olmsted County, Minnesota. Mayo Clin Proc 78(2): 161.

Carey, J, Weintraub, A. 2007 Aug 7. When medical studies collide: Contradictory reports? Meta-analysis may make things more confusing. BusinessWeek.

Flora, C. Sleep the fat off: Lose weight while you sleep. <www.PsychologyToday.com>. Accessed Oct 2008.

Olshansky, SJ, Passaro, DJ, Hershow, RC, Layden, J, Carnes, BA, Brody, J, Hayflick, L, Butler, RN, Allison, DB, Ludwig, DS. 2007. A potential decline in life expectancy in the United States in the 21st century. NEJM 352(11): 1138–1145.

Preston, SH. 2005. Deadweight? The influence of obesity on longevity. NEJM 352(11): 1135–1137.

Taheri, S, Lin, L, Austin, D, Young, T, Mignot, E. 2004. Short sleep duration is associated with reduced leptin, elevated ghrelin, and increased body mass index. PLoS Med 1(3): e62.

Traub, M. 2005. Statistically significant: Is scientific evidence really enough? Bottom Line's Daily Health News. <www.bottomlinesecrets.com>. Accessed Oct 2008.

Turner, RB, Bauer, R, Woelkart, K, Hulsey, TC, Gangemi, JD. 2005. An evaluation of echinacea angustifolia in experimental rhinovirus infections. NEJM 353 (4): 341–348.

Von Bubnoff, A. 2007 17 Sep. Scientists do the numbers. Los Angeles Times. <www.articles.latimes.com>. Accessed Oct 2008.

Wang, Y, Beydoun, MA, Liang, L, Caballero, B, Kumanyika, SK. 2008. Will all Americans become overweight or obese? Estimating the progression and cost of the U.S. obesity epidemic. Obesity: 16(10): 2323–2330.

Chapter 2: Our Compromised Immune System

Baker, L. 2004 Sep 30. Research findings continue to support chronic cellular inflammation as precursor of heart disease, diabetes. UB Reporter. <www.buffalo.edu/ubreporter/archives>. Accessed Oct 2008.

Chandra, RK. 1997. Nutrition and the immune system: An introduction. Am J Clin Nutr 66(2): 460S–463S.

Clays, E, DeBacquer, D, Delanghe, J, Kittel, F, Renterghem, L, De Backer, G. 2005. Associations between dimensions of job stress and biomarkers of inflammation and infection. J Occup Env Med 47(9): 878–883.

Fontana, L, Eagon, JC, Trujillo, ME, Scherer, PE, Klein, S. 2007. Visceral fat adipokine secretion is associated with systemic inflammation in obese humans. Diabetes 56(4): 1010-1013.

Gangwisch, JE, Heymsfield, SB, et al. 2006. Short sleep duration as a risk factor for hypertension: Analyses of the first national health and nutrition examination survey. Hypertension 47: 833–839.

Ghanim, H, Aljada, A, Dandona, P, et al. 2004. Circulating mononuclear cells in the obese are in a proinflammatory state. Circulation 110: 1564–1571.

Heptinstall, S, May, J, et al. 2006. Cocoa flavanols and platelet and leukocyte function: Recent in vitro and ex vivo studies in healthy adults. J Cardio Pharm 47 (suppl 2): S197–S205.

Shade, ED, Ulrich, CM, et al. 2004. Frequent intentional weight loss is associated with lower natural killer cell cyto-toxicity in postmenopausal women: Possible long-term immune effects. J Am Diet Assoc 104(6): 892–894.

Chapter 3: Oxidation, Aging, and Disease

Dockery, DW, Stone, PH. 2005. Cardiovascular risks from fine particulate air pollution. NEJM 356(5): 511–513.

Grandjean, P, Landrigan, PJ. 2006. Developmental neuro-toxicity of industrial chemicals. The Lancet 368(9553): 2167–2178.

Liu, RH. 2003. Health benefits of fruit and vegetables are from additive and synergistic combinations of phytochemicals. Am J Clin Nutr 78 (suppl): 517S–20S.

Tosca, L, Zern, TL, Fernandez, ML. 2005. Cardioprotective effects of dietary polyphenols. J of Nutr 35(10): 2291–2294.

Chapter 4: Wellness vs. Illness: The Road to Optimum Health

Bennett, RM. 1999. Emerging concepts in the neurobiology of chronic pain: Evidence of abnormal sensory processing in fibromyalgia. Mayo Clin Proc 74(4): 385–98.

Bennett, RM. 1998. Disordered growth hormone secretion in fibromyalgia: A review of recent findings ad a hypothesizing etiology. Z Rheumatol 57(S2): 72–76.

Goldenberg, DL, et al. 2004. Management of fibromyalgia syn-drome. JAMA 292(19): 2388–2395.

Limer, KL, Nicholl, BI, et al. 2008. Exploring the genetic susceptibility of chronic widespread pain: The tender points in genetic association studies. Rheumatology 47(5): 572–577.

Nielson, WR, Jensen, MP. 2004. Relationship between changes in coping and treatment outcome in patients with fibromyalgia syndrome. Pain 109(3): 233–241.

Physical activity and good nutrition: Essential elements to prevent chronic diseases and obesity. National Center for Chronic Disease Prevention and Health Promotion (CDC), 2004.

Pollan, M. 2007 Jan 28. Unhappy meals. The New York Times Magazine. 40-69.

Rader, A. 2007. Real food vs. nutritionism: How food science has failed us. Acupuncture Today 08(04). <www.acupuncturetoday.com>. Accessed Nov 2008.

Vasan, RS, Beiser, A, et al. 2002. Residual lifetime risk for developing hypertension in middle-aged women and men: The Framingham heart study. JAMA 287: 1003–1010.

Chapter 5: Eating Well and Enjoying It

Abuissa, H, O'Keefe, JH, Cordain, L. 2005. Realigning our 21st century diet and lifestyle with our hunter-gatherer genetic identity. Dir Psych 25: SR1–SR10.

Clemens, RA, Coughlin, J. 2007. Coffee and health: Surprisingly good news. Food Tech 61: 17.

Clement, LP, Scimeca, JA, Thompson, HJ. 1994. Conjugated linoleic acid. A powerful anticarcinogen from animal fat sources. Cancer 74 (S3): 1050–1054.

Cordain L, Eaton, SB, Brand-Miller, J, Mann, N, Hill, K. 2002. The paradoxical nature of hunter-gatherer diets: Meat based, yet non-atherogenic. Eur J Clin Nutr 56 (suppl 1): S42–S52.

Cordain, L, Lindeberg, S, Hurtado, M, Hill, K, Eaton, SB, Brand-Miller, J. 2002. Acne vulgaris: A disease of western civilization. Arch Dermatol 138: 1584–90.

Douglas, J. 2003. Nature's perfect food: Discover the amazing health benefits of the fruit from the Amazon's "tree of life." Health Sciences Institute. <www.hsibaltimore.com>. Accessed Dec 2009.

Eat your fruits and vegetables: One extra serving per day may lower your risk of head and neck cancer. ScienceDaily. <www.sciencedaily.com>. Accessed Oct 2008.

Eaton, S, Konner, M. 1985. Paleolithic nutrition: A consideration of its nature and current implications. NEJM 312: 283–289.

Eaton, SB, Strassman, BI, et al. 2002. Evolutionary health promotion. Prev Med 34: 109–118.

Einbond, LS, Reynertson, KA, et al. 2004. Anthocyanin antioxidants from edible fruits. Food Chem 84: 23–28.

Gould, KS. 2004. Nature's Swiss Army knife: The diverse protective roles of anthocyanins in leaves. J Biom & Biot 5: 314–320.

Graham, T. 2003. The fruit that packs a punch. Men's Journal. <www.mensjournal.com>. Accessed Nov 2008.

Higdon, JV, Frei, B. 2006. Coffee and health: A review of recent human research. Crit Rev Food Sci Nutr 46(2): 101–123.

Hoyt, G, Hickey, MS, Cordain, L. 2005. Dissociation of the glycaemic and insulinaemic responses to whole and skimmed milk. Br J Nutr 93: 175–177.

Lichtenthaler, R, Rodrigues, RB, et al. 2005. Total oxidant scavenging capacities of Euterpe oleracea Mart (acai). Int J Food Sci Nutr 56(1): 53–64.

Lindeberg, S, Cordain, L, Eaton, SB. 2003. Biological and clinical potential of a Paleolithic diet. J Nutri Environ Med 13(3): 149–160.

O'Keefe, JH Jr, Cordain, L. 2004. Cardiovascular disease resulting from a diet and lifestyle at odds with our Paleolithic genome: How to become a 21st-century hunter-gatherer. Mayo Clin Proc 79(1): 101–8.

Pederson, DJ, Lessard, SJ, et al. 2008. High rates of muscle glycogen resynthesis after exhaustive exercise when carbo-hydrate is co-ingested with caffeine. J of App Phys 105: 7–13.

Sebastian, A, Frassetto, LA, et al. 2002. Estimation of the net acid load of the diet of ancestral preagricultural Homo sapiens and their hominid ancestors. Am J Clin Nutr 76(6): 1308–16.

Ward, C. The perils of nutritionism: Or, how the food industry pimped my breakfast. Catalyst Magazine. <www.catalaystmagazine.net>. Accessed Dec 2008.

Wu, H, Feng, L. 2006. Abstract 1367: T cell accumulation in adipose tissue in obesity-related insulin resistance induced by a high-fat diet. Circulation 11(4:II): 260.

Chapter 6: Supplement Your Health

Arehart-Treichel, J. 2002. Can taking supplements help curb prison violence? Psyc News 37(19): 26.

Carr, AC, Frei, B. 1999. Toward a new recommended dietary allowance for vitamin C based on antioxidant and health effects in humans. Am J Clin Nutr 69(6): 1086–1107.

Fletcher, RH, Fairfield, KM. 2002. Vitamins for chronic disease prevention in adults. JAMA 287: 3127–3129.

Gesch, B, Hammond, S, Hampson, S, et al. 2002. Influence of supplementary vitamins, minerals, and essential fatty acids on the antisocial behaviour of young adult prisoners. Brit J Psy-chiatry 181: 22–8.

Jacob, RA, Sotoudeh, G. 2002. Vitamin C function and status in chronic disease. Nutr Clin Care 5(2): 47–49.

Chapter 7: Exercise and Wellness

Duncan, GE, Perri, MG, et al. 2003. Exercise training, without weight loss, increases insulin sensitivity and postheparin plasma lipase activity in previously sedentary adults. Diab Care 26: 557–562.

Ebersole, KE, Dugas, LR, et al. 2008. Energy expenditure and adiposity in Nigerian and African-American women. Obesity 16(9): 2148–2154.

Lane, AM, Lovejoy, DJ. 2001. The effects of exercise on mood changes: The moderating effect of depressed mood. J Sport Med Phys Fit 41(04): 539.

Lemura, LM, von Duvillard, SP, Mookerjee, S. 2000. The effects of physical training of functional capacity in adults. Ages 46 to 90: a meta-analysis. J Sport Med Phys Fit 40(01): 1.

Chapter 8: Stress Management

Anderson, JW, Liu, C, Kryscio, RJ, 2008. Blood pressure response to Transcendental Meditation: A meta-analysis. Amer J Hypertension 21: 310–316.

Barnes, VA, Treiber, FA, Davis, H. 2001. Impact of Transcendental Meditation on cardiovascular function at rest and during acute stress in adolescents with high normal blood pressure. J Psychosom Res 51(4): 597–605.

Always on my mind: Britons are making themselves ill with worry. (Press Release), Bupa Insurance, 2007 Nov 19. <www.bupa.co.uk/health>. Accessed Jan 2009.

Epel, ES, Lin, J, Wilhelm, FH, et al. 2006. Cell aging in relation to stress arousal and cardiovascular disease risk factors. Psychoneuro 21(3): 277–87.

Paul-Labrador, M, Polk, D, et al. 2006. Effects of a randomized controlled trial of Transcendental Meditation on components of the metabolic syndrome in subjects with coronary heart disease. Arch Intern Med 166: 1218–1224.

Chapter 9: A Healthy Brain

Durga, J, Morris, MC, Tangney, CC. 2007. Is dietary intake of folate too low? Lancet 369(9557): 166–167.

Downard, B. 2008. Food for thought: Cognition nutrition: Eat your way to a better brain. Economist. <www.economist.com>. Accessed Oct 2008.

Gómez-Pinilla, F. 2008. Brain foods: The effects of nutrients on brain function. Nat Rev Neurosci 9(7): 568–578.

Harburger, LL, Chinonyere K, et al. 2007. Single enrichment variables differentially reduce age-related memory decline in female mice. Behav Neuro 121(4): 679-688.

Stein, J, Schettler, T. 2008. Environmental threats to healthy aging. Greater Boston Physicians for Social Responsibility and Science and Environmental Health.

Wang, HX, Karp, A, et al. 2009. Personality and lifestyle in relation to dementia incidence. Neurology 72: 253–259.

Chapter 10: Aging on Your Own Terms

Manson, JE, Allison, MA, et al. 2007. Estrogen therapy and coronary artery calcification. NEJM 356(25): 2591–2602.

Minor, MA. 1996. Arthritis and exercise: The times they are a-changin'. Arth & Rheum 9(2): 79–81.

Villareal, DT, Fontana, L, et al. 2006. Bone mineral density response to caloric restriction–induced weight loss or exercise-induced weight loss: A randomized controlled trial. Arch Intern Med 166: 2502–2510.

Chapter 11: Looking Your Best

Beyer, AM. 2008. Beauty from the inside out. Inside Cosmeceuticals. <www.insidecosmeceuticals.com>. Accessed Nov 2008.

Biesalski HK, Obermueller-Jevic, UC. 2001. UV light, beta-carotene and human skin: Beneficial and potentially harmful effects. Arch Biochem Biophys 389(1): 1–6.

Boelsma, E, Hendriks, HFJ, Roza, L. 2001. Nutritional skin care: Health effects of micronutrients and fatty acids. Am J Clin Nutr 73: 853–64.

Cordain L. 2006. Dietary implications for the development of acne: A shifting paradigm. U.S. Dermatology Review. London: Touch Briefings Publications.

Does nutrition make a difference in skin rejuvenation? <Smartskincare.com>. Accessed Oct 2008.

Edelberg, D. Supplement recommendations for skin health. <www.
WholeHealthMD.com>. Accessed Oct 2008.

Fisher, GJ, Wang, ZQ. 1997. Pathophysiology of premature skin aging
induced by ultraviolet light. NEJM 337(20): 1463–1465.

Fuchs, J, Kern, H. 1998. Modulation of UV-light-induced skin inflammation by d-alpha-tocopherol and L-ascorbic acid: A clinical study using solar
simulated radiation. Free Radic Biol Med 25(9): 1006–1012.

Henderson, A. 1996. Skin, aging & treatment. Women's Health Weekly
(N): 19.

Hyland, P. 2008. All about wrinkles. <www.Health.Discovery.com>. Accessed
Oct 2008.

Landsmann, MA. 2006. Healthy skin, naturally. Healthy Aging. <www.
advanceweb.com/healthyaging>. Accessed Nov 2008.

Lee, J, Jiang, S, Levine, N, Watson, RR. 2000. Carotenoid supplementation
reduces erythema in human skin after simulated solar radiation exposure. Proc
Soc Exp Biol Med 223(2): 170–174.

Lin, YL, Selim, MA, et al. 2003. UV photoprotection by combination topical
antioxidants vitamin C and vitamin E. J Amer Acad Derm 48(6): 866–874.

McDaniel, D. 2006. A radical new approach to anti-aging. Cosmetic Surgery
Times. <cosmeticsurgery-times.modernmedicine.com>. Accessed Nov 2008.

Mitsuishi, T, Shimoda, T. The effects of topical application of phy-
tonadione, retinol, and vitamins C and E on infraorbital dark circles and
wrinkles of the lower eyelids. J Cosm Derm. Apr 2004; 3(2): 73–75.

Murray, JC, Burch, JA. 2008. A topical antioxidant solution containing vitamins
C and E stabilized by ferulic acid provides protection for human skin against
damage caused by ultraviolet irradiation. J Amer Acad Derm 59(3): 418–425.

Placzek, M, Gaube, S, et al. 2005. Ultraviolet B-induced DNA damage in
human epidermis is modified by the antioxidants ascorbic acid and d-tocoph-
erol. J Inv Derm 124(2): 304–307.

Rorie, S. 2008. A youthful pursuit with antioxidants. Inside Cosmeceuticals. <www.insidecosmeceuticals.com>. Accessed Nov 2008.

Stahl, W, Heinrich, U, Jungmann, H, Sies, H, Tronnier, 2000. H. Carotenoids and carotenoids plus vitamin E protect against ultraviolet light-induced erythema in humans. Am J Clin Nutr 71(3): 795–798.

Stukin, S. 2007. Will taking a pill achieve beautiful skin? Los Angeles Times. <www.articles.latimes.com>. Accessed Nov 2008.

Treloar, V, Logan, AC, Danby, FW, Cordain, L, Mann, NJ. 2008. Comment on acne and glycemic index. J Am Acad Dermatol 58(1): 175–177.

Verma, SBB, Draelos, ZD. 2008. Cosmetic dermatology versus cosmetology: A misnomer in need of urgent correction. Indian J Derm, Ven Lep 74(2): 92–93.

Wright, R. 2008. Antiaging: Beauty and beyond. Neutraceutical World. <www.neutraceuticalworld.com>. Accessed Nov 2008.

Books

Abramson, J. 2004. Overdosed America. New York: Harper Collins.

Cordain, L. 2002. The Paleo diet: Lose weight and get healthy by eating the food you were designed to eat. New York: John Wiley and Sons.

Cordain L. 2006. Implications of Plio-Pleistocene Hominin diets for modern humans. In early Hominin diets: The known, the unknown, and the unknowable. New York: Oxford University Press.

Cordain L. 2006. Saturated fat consumption in ancestral human diets: Implications for contemporary intakes. Phytochemicals, Nutrient-Gene Interactions. Boca Raton, FL: CRC Press (Taylor & Francis Group).

Eaton SB, Cordain L, Sebastian A. 2007. The ancestral biomedical environment in endothelial biomedicine. New York: Cambridge University Press.

Erasmus, U. 1993. Fats that heal, fats that kill. Bumaby BC, Canada: Alive Books.

Packer, L. 2006. Antioxidant food supplements in human health. New York: Academic Press.

Pollan, M. 2006. The omnivore's dilemma. New York: Penguin Press.

Mercola, J. 2007. Take control of your health, Schaumberg, IL: Mercola.com.

Murray, M. 1998. Encyclopedia of natural medicine (revised 2nd edition). New York: Three Rivers Press..

Murray, M. 1996. Encyclopedia of nutritional supplements. Rocklin, CA: Prima Publishing.

Murray, M. 1994. Natural alternatives to over-the-counter and prescription drugs. New York: William Morrow and Co.

Nestle, M. 2002. Food politics. Berkeley, CA: University of California Press.

Robins, N. 2005. Copeland's cure. New York: Alfred A. Knopf.

Roizen, MF, Oz, MC. 2005. You: The owner's manual. New York: Harper Collins.

Schapiro, M. 2007. Exposed: The toxic chemistry of everyday products and what's at stake for American power. White River Junction, VT: Chelsea Green Publishing.

Organizations

Agency for Healthcare Research and Quality (HHS)
Rockville, MD
www.ahrq.gov

Alzheimer's Association
Chicago, IL
www.alz.org

American Academy of Dermatology (AAD)
Schaumburg, IL
www.aad.org

American Association of Naturopathic Physicians (AANP)
Washington, D.C.
www.naturopathic.org

American Botanical Council (ABC)
Austin, TX
www.herbalgram.org

American Cancer Society
Atlanta, GA
www.cancer.org

American Chronic Pain Association
Rocklin, CA
www.theacpa.org

American College of Allergy,
Asthma, and Immunology
Arlington Heights, IL
www.acaai.org

American College of
Gastroenterology (ACG)
Arlington, VA
www.acg.gi.org

American College of Rheumatology
(Arthritis and Rheumatism)
Atlanta, GA
http://www.rheumatology.org

The American College of Sports
Medicine (ACSM)
Indianapolis, IN
www.acsm.org

American Council on Exercise
San Diego, CA
www.acefitness.org

American Council for Fitness and
Nutrition
Washington, D.C.
www.acfn.org

American Diabetes Association
Alexandria, VA
www.diabetes.org

American Dietetic Association
Chicago, IL
www.eatright.org

American Gastroenterological
Association
Bethesda, MD
www.gastro.org

American Heart Association
Dallas, TX
www.americanheart.org

Arthritis Foundation
Atlanta, GA
www.arthritis.org

The Center for Mindfulness
in Medicine, Health Care, and
Society (CFM)
Boston, MA
www.umassmed.edu/content.
aspx?id=41252

Centers for Disease Control and
Prevention
Atlanta, GA
www.cdc.gov

CenterWatch
Boston, MA
www.centerwatch.com

Environmental Protection Agency
(EPA)
Washington, D.C.
www.epa.gov

European Prospective Investigation
into Cancer and Nutrition (EPIC)
Lyon, France
epic.iarc.fr

Food and Drug Administration
(FDA)
Rockville, MD
www.fda.gov

Harvard Center for Cancer
Prevention
Cambridge, MA
harvardscience.harvard.edu

Healthy People 2010
Office of Disease Prevention and
Health Promotion
Department of Health and Human
Services (HHS)
Rockville, MD
www.healthypeople.gov

MacArthur Foundation Research
Network on Successful Aging
Columbia University
New York, NY
www.agingsocietynetwork.org/about

Mayo Clinic
Rochester, MN
www.mayoclinic.com

MetLife Foundation
New York, NY
www.metlife.com

Morehouse School of Medicine
Atlanta, GA
MSM.edu

National Cancer Institute
Bethesda, MD
www.cancer.gov

National Heart, Lung, and Blood
Institute
Bethesda, MD
www.nhlbi.nih.gov/whi

National Institute on Aging (NIA-
NIH)
Bethesda, MD
www.nia.nih.gov

National Institute of Neurological
Disorders and Stroke (NINDS-NIH)
Bethesda, MD
www.ninds.nih.gov

New England Centenarian Study
www.bumc.bu.edu/centenarian

Office of Complementary Medicine
(NIH)
Gaithersburg, MD
nccam.nih.gov

The Okinawa Centenarian Study
www.okicent.org

OneWorld Health
San Francisco, CA
www.oneworldhealth.org

Productive Aging Laboratory
Dallas, TX
agingmind.utdallas.edu

Rice University
Houston, TX
www.rice.edu

Rush University Medical Center
Chicago, IL
www.rush.edu

The Sleep Foundation
Washington, D.C.
www.sleepfoundation.org

Tufts University School of Nutrition
Science and Policy
Boston, MA
nutrition.tufts.edu

U.S. Department of Agriculture
(USDA)
Washington, D.C.
www.usda.gov

University of Pennsylvania School of
Medicine
Philadelphia, PA
www.med.upenn.edu